# Operating Department Practice
# A–Z

# Operating Department Practice A–Z

**Edited by**

## Brian Smith
Dip. Psych., Cert. Ed., FAETC, RODP
*Senior Lecturer, Continual Professional Development*
*Formerly*
*Senior Lecturer, ODP Education*
*Edge Hill College of Higher Education*


## Tom Williams
M.Phil., BA, Dip. Ed., Cert. Ed., FAETC,
Dip. (HSM), Dip. (IOSH), RODP, Dip. IOTT.
*Senior Lecturer, ODP Education*
*Edge Hill College of Higher Education*
*Formerly*
*Senior Lecturer,*
*West Midlands ODP Education Centre and*
*Principal, ODP Training Programme*
*Riyadh Al Kharj Armed Forces Hospitals, Saudi Arabia*

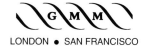

LONDON • SAN FRANCISCO

A 042343

© 2004

Greenwich Medical Media Limited
137 Euston Road
London NW1 2AA

870 Market Street, Ste 720,
San Francisco, CA 94102

ISBN 1 84110 1931

First Published 2004

WO 500

A catalogue record for this book is available from the British Library.

Project Manager
Gill Clark

Typeset by Charon Tec Pvt. Ltd, Chennai, India

Printed in the UK by the Cromwell Press

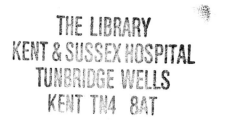

# Contents

# Preface

Within the hospital setting the operating department is as unique as any other. Therefore, due to its specialised and diverse activities the terminology used will inevitably be specialised and dedicated to tasks performed and the role of the staff.

With this in mind, the decision was made to provide a reference source in the form of a dictionary that deals not only with standard medical/surgical terms and words but additional jargon that has become an everyday part of perioperative terminology.

Many allied professions have similar text pertaining specifically to their environment and roles, however no such publication is available that exclusively deals with the operating department and its activities. Hence, the production of this book.

It is targeted primarily at student ODPs, those undergoing further training: and existing theatre staff to use as an aid and reference source. It is hoped that student nurses, medical students, junior doctors, surgical ward staff and other colleagues in related departments of X-ray, physiotherapy, bio-engineering/medical physics, medical secretaries, etc. will find the text of value when needing to relate to theatres.

The authors and publisher would welcome submissions, suggestions or any constructive comments towards future editions, please contact us by email via the publishers at gnuttall@cambridge.org.

*T. Williams*
*B. Smith*
Liverpool, 2004

# Contributors

## Main contributors

Tom Williams
*Senior Lecturer*
*Edge Hill College of*
  *Higher Education*
*Liverpool*

Brian Smith
*Senior Lecturer*
*Edge Hill College of*
  *Higher Education*
*Liverpool*

Jean Hinton
*Senior Lecturer*
*Edge Hill College of*
  *Higher Education*
*Liverpool*

Josie Williams
*Senior Lecturer*
*Edge Hill College of*
  *Higher Education*
*Liverpool*

## Additional contributors

Paul Wicker
*Programme Leader*
*Edge Hill College of*
  *Higher Education*
*Liverpool*

Cheryl Wayne
*Senior Lecturer*
*Edge Hill College of*
  *Higher Education*
*Liverpool*

Rita Hehir
*Senior Lecturer*
*Edge Hill College of*
  *Higher Education*
*Liverpool*

Jill McKeen
*Senior Lecturer*
*Edge Hill College of*
  *Higher Education*
*Liverpool*

Also thanks to the following Edge Hill ODP students for their contributions:

Kevin Murphy
Sandra Fox
Robert J. Mitchell
Neil Herbert

# Foreword

One of the greatest pleasures of my professional life has been observing the development of the operating department practitioner (ODP) grade. I trained in anaesthesia in Liverpool, UK, in an environment where operating department assistants (ODAs) were respected members of the theatre team. They were well established in this area, mainly because enterprising consultant anaesthetists had trained them to the highest standards, teaching them skills in emergency medicine and anaesthesia of which many a houseman would be justifiably proud today. Examples would include: Dr AA Gilbertson at Sefton General Hospital, Liverpool, who trained one of the main authors of this book, Tom Williams; Dr RS Ahearn at the Northern Hospital, Liverpool; Dr THL Bryson at Liverpool Women's Hospital; and Drs Colin Ince and Norton Williams at Whiston Hospital, Merseyside, where the other main author of this book, Brian Smith, worked.

By their example, anaesthetists such as these set high standards for ODAs to achieve. They gave the ODAs that essential professionalism which made them a pivotal part of the operating department team. Much was demanded of these ODAs in terms of time and effort, but in reward they received the unswerving support of the anaesthetic fraternity. Generations of anaesthetists came to respect them, and I proudly include myself in these minions. In addition, their unique Liverpool humour made these men (and they were mainly men at that time), loved by us all. It is apposite that increasing numbers of women (many of whom are qualified nurses), are now training as ODPs, and this is reflected in the strong female contribution to this book, which is also satisfying to observe.

There was no formal career structure for ODAs 30 years ago. It is only in the last 25 years that formal teaching has become established nationally for these essential workers, and now the ODP in training undergoes a structured programme of classroom as well as practical teaching. The standard of theoretical knowledge required of them to complete this training is very high indeed, and would surprise many unwitting medical practitioners.

This dictionary will contribute significantly to the trainee's comprehension of operating theatre life. Its structured approach makes for easy access and understanding, and it is most comprehensive in its detail. The reader is even told phonetically how to say each of the listed words. (Anaesthetists and nurses too may find this facility useful!) Equipment, drugs, diseases, symptoms, signs, anatomy, operations, and even theatre slang are covered. At the end a list of useful websites, and some normal physiological values are also included.

I am enormously proud to have watched these authors develop into significant academic contributors to their profession. I congratulate them wholeheartedly on their achievement, and very much hope that they continue to make such a major contribution in the future, for this is just what their own (strict) teachers would have expected.

Jennifer M. Hunter
*Professor of Anaesthesia,*
*University of Liverpool*

*Editor-in-Chief*
*British Journal of Anaesthesia*

*February 2004*

# Acknowledgements

The idea for this book came from a realisation that although numerous medical-related resources already exist, there was nothing available that contributed directly to the role of Operating Department Staff. Therefore, it is envisaged that this text will supplement the wealth of information contained in alternative dictionaries but with an emphasis towards peri-operative practice.

We would like to thank all colleagues, students, clinical staff who have assisted with contributions and ideas; also, ODP Centre Secretary, Karen Williams, for IT advice and assistance.

Also thanks and appreciation to Professor J. Hunter for agreeing to write the Foreword for the book and provide expert and invaluable advice.

*T. Williams*
*B. Smith*
Liverpool, 2004

# Medical terminology

## Prefixes, suffixes and roots

| | |
|---|---|
| a-, an- | not, without |
| ab- | away from |
| ad- | towards |
| aden(o)- | gland |
| adip- | fat |
| aemia | blood |
| aesthesia | sensation |
| algia | pain |
| angi(o)- | blood vessel |
| ante- | before, in front |
| anti- | against |
| arthr(o)- | joint |
| asis | state of |
| audio- | hearing, sound |
| andro- | man |
| auto- | self |
| bi-, bis- | two |
| bil- | bile |
| blephar(o)- | eyelid |
| brachi(o)- | arm |
| brady- | slow |
| bronch(o)- | windpipe |
| carcin- | cancer |
| cardio | heart |
| carp- | wrist |
| centi- | a hundredth |
| cephal(o)- | head |
| cerebr(o)- | brain |
| cervic(o)- | neck |
| chemo- | chemical |
| chol- | bile |
| chondr-o | cartilage |

| | |
|---|---|
| co-, col-, com-, con- | together, with |
| colp- | vagina |
| contra- | against, counter, e.g. drug |
| cost(o)- | rib |
| costal | relating to the rib |
| crani(o)- | skull |
| cryo- | cold |
| cyst | bladder |
| cyt- | cell |
| dacry- | tear |
| dactyl- | finger |
| dent- | tooth |
| derm- | skin |
| di-, diplo- | two, double |
| dia- | through |
| diplo- | double |
| dis- | apart, away from |
| dors- | back |
| dys- | difficult, abnormal |
| ect- | outside |
| ectomy | cutting out |
| em-, en-, end-, ent- | in, inside, within |
| endo- | within, intp |
| enter(o)- | intestine |
| epi- | upon, over |
| eu- | good, normal |
| ex-, exo- | out of |
| ferro(i)- | iron |
| gastr- | stomach |
| genito- | genitals |
| gingivo- | gums |
| glosso- | tongue |
| glyco- | sugar |
| gynae | women |
| haem- | blood |
| hecta- | one hundred |
| hemi- | half |
| hepat- | liver |
| hetero- | unlike, dissimilar |
| hidro- | sweat |
| hist- | tissue, web |
| homeo- | like |
| hydro- | water |
| hygro- | moisture |
| hyper- | above |

| | |
|---|---|
| hypno- | sleep |
| hypo- | below |
| hyster(o)- | womb or uterus |
| idio- | peculiar to, own |
| immuno- | immunity or immune |
| infra- | below |
| inter- | between |
| intra- | within |
| intro- | inwards |
| iso- | equal |
| -itis | inflammation |
| kilo- | one thousand |
| lacto- | milk |
| laparo- | loins or abdomen |
| laryng(o)- | windpipe (upper) and larynx |
| later-o | side |
| leuc-, leuk- | white |
| lipo- | fat |
| lith(o)- | stone |
| lordo- | bent forward |
| macro- | large |
| mal- | poor, abnormal |
| mano- | pressure |
| mast- | breast |
| medi- | middle |
| mega- | big, enlarged |
| meso- | middle |
| micr- | small |
| micro- | one millionth |
| milli- | thousandth |
| mono- | single |
| mort- | death |
| multi- | many |
| myelo- | marrow |
| myo- | muscle |
| narco- | sleep, stupor |
| naso- | nose |
| neo- | new |
| nephr(o)- | kidney |
| neur(o)- | nerve |
| nulli- | none |
| odont- | tooth |
| oligo- | difficult |
| oma- | tumour |
| onco- | tumour |

| | |
|---|---|
| oophoro- | ovary |
| -opsy | looking |
| opthalm(o)- | eye |
| orchid- | testis |
| os-, oste- | bone |
| -ostomy | opening |
| -otomy | cutting |
| paed- | child |
| pan- | all |
| para- | next to, adjacent |
| patho- | disease |
| per- | through |
| peri- | around |
| -pexy | fixing |
| phleb(o)- | vein |
| pneum(o)- | lung |
| poly- | many |
| post- | after |
| pre- | before, infront of |
| primi- | first |
| proct- | anus |
| proximo- | near |
| pseudo- | false |
| psycho- | mind |
| pyo- | pus, matter |
| pyr- | heat, fever, fire |
| retro- | backwards |
| rhin(o)- | nose |
| -rrhaphy | repair |
| salping- | uterine tube |
| sclero- | hard |
| -scopy | looking |
| semi- | half |
| sub- | below |
| super- | above |
| supra- | above |
| tachy- | quick |
| thoraco- | chest |
| thromb- | clot |
| -tome | cutting instrument |
| trans- | through, across |
| ultra- | beyond |
| uni- | one |
| uri- | uric acid |
| vas/vaso- | duct or blood vessel |

| | |
|---|---|
| veno- | vein |
| ventro- | front |
| vesic- | vesicle |
| zym- | enzyme, fermentation |

# Abbreviations

| | |
|---|---|
| AAA | Triple A – Abdominal Aortic Aneurysm |
| ABG | Arterial blood gases |
| ACLS | Advanced Cardiac Life Support |
| ADH | Anti Diuretic Hormone |
| AIDS | Acquired immune deficiency syndrome |
| AKU | Artificial kidney unit |
| ALERT | Acute Life-Threatening Events Recognition and Treatment |
| AODP | Association of Operating Department Practitioners |
| APH | Ante Partum Haemorrhage |
| ARC | AIDS Related Complex |
| ARDS | Adult respiratory distress syndrome |
| ASA | American Society of Anesthesiologists |
| ASD | Atrial Septal Defect |
| ASP | Advanced Scrub Practitioner |
| ATLS | Advanced Trauma Life Support |
| BAHA | Bone anchored hearing aid |
| BAWO | Bilateral antrum washout |
| BCC | Basal cell carcinoma |
| BCLS | Basic Cardiac Life Support |
| BD | Twice daily |
| BID | Brought in dead |
| BIPP | Bisthmus iodine paraffin paste |
| BKA | Below knee amputation |
| BP | Blood pressure |
| Bx | Biopsy |
| C5 | Fifth cervical vertebra |
| Ca | Carcinoma |
| CABG | Coronary Artery Bypass Graft |
| CAT | Computed axial tomography |
| CBD | Common bile duct |
| CCF | Congestive cardiac failure |
| CCU | Coronary Care Unit |
| CDH | Cogenital Dislocation of Hip |

| | |
|---|---|
| CHOLE | Cholecystectomy |
| CICU | Coronary Intensive Care Unit |
| CNS | Central nervous system |
| $CO_2$ | Carbon dioxide |
| COAD | Chronic obstructive airways disease |
| COPD | Chronic obstructive pulmonary disease |
| COSHH | Control of substances hazardous to health |
| CPAP | Continuous positive airway pressure |
| CPR | Cardiopulmonary resuscitation |
| CRF | Chronic Renal Failure |
| CS | Caesarean Section |
| CSF | Cerebrospinal fluid |
| CSSD | Central Sterile Services Department |
| CVA | Cerebrovascular accident |
| CVP | Central venous pressure |
| CVS | Cardiovascular system |
| CXR | Chest X-ray |
| D&C | Dilatation and curettage |
| D&V | Diarrhoea & Vomiting |
| DCIA | Deep circumflex iliac artery |
| DCP | Dynamic compression plate |
| DCS | Dynamic compression screw |
| DHS | Dynamic hip screw |
| DIC | Disseminated intravascular coagulation |
| DNA | Did not arrive |
| DNR | Do Not Resuscitate |
| DOA | Dead on arrival |
| DPT | Diphtheria, Tetanus, Pertussis (triple vaccine) |
| DU | Duodenal ulcer |
| DVT | Deep vein thrombosis |
| EBME | Electrical Biomedical Engineering |
| ECF | Extracellular fluid |
| ECG | Electrocardiography |
| ECT | Electroconvulsive therapy |
| EEG | Electroencephalogram |
| ENT | Ear, nose and throat |
| ERCP | Endoscopic retrograde cholangiopancreatography |
| ERPC | Evacuation of retained products of conception |
| ESR | Erythrocyte Sedimentation Rate |
| ESWL | Extracorporeal Shock Wave Lithotripsy |
| ETT | Endotracheal tube |
| EUA | Examinations under anaesthetic |
| EWA | Examination without anaesthetic |
| FB | Foreign Body |
| FBC | Full blood count |

| | |
|---|---|
| FBS | Fasting Blood Sugar |
| FESS | Functional endoscopic sinus surgery |
| FEV | Forced expiratory volume |
| FFP | Fresh frozen plasma |
| FGF | Fresh Gas Flow |
| FNAB | Fine needle aspiration biopsy |
| FRC | Functional residual capacity |
| FS | Frozen section |
| FSH | Follicle stimulating hormone |
| FVC | Forced vital capacity |
| GA | General anaesthesia |
| GCS | Glasgow coma scale |
| GI | Gastro Intestinal |
| GIFT | Gamete Intra Fallopian Transfer |
| GIT | Gastrointestinal tract |
| Grav (I, II, III) | Number of pregnancies |
| GSS | Group and save serum |
| GTN | Glyceral trinitrate |
| GU | Genito Urinary |
| HAS | Human albumin solutions |
| HASAWA | Health and Safety At Work Act |
| Hb | Haemaglobin |
| HBV | Hepatitis B Virus |
| HCA | Health care assistant |
| HDU | High dependency unit |
| HIV | Human immunodeficiency virus |
| HNPU | Has not passed urine |
| HPC | Health Professions Council |
| ICF | Intra Cellular Fluid |
| ICP | Intracranial pressure |
| ICU | Intensive care unit |
| IM | Intramuscularly |
| IO | Intra Ocular |
| IOL | Intraoccular lens |
| IPPR | Intermittent Positive Pressure Respiration |
| IPPV | Intermittent positive pressure ventilation |
| IR | Infrared |
| IUCD | Intra Uterine Contraceptive Device |
| IV | Intravenous |
| IVF | In Vitro Fertilisation |
| IVP | Intra Venous Pyelogram |
| IVU | Intravenous urography |
| KCL | Potassium chloride |
| KUB | Kidney Ureter Bladder |
| LA | Local anaesthetic |

**Operating Department Practice A–Z**

| | |
|---|---|
| LAFP | Left Atrial Filling Pressure |
| LASER | Light amplification by simulated emission of radiation |
| LAVH | Laparoscopically Assisted Vaginal Hysterectomy |
| LFA | Low Friction Arthroplasty |
| LIF | Left ileac fossa |
| LIH | Left Inguinal Hernia |
| LMA | Laryngeal Mask Airway |
| LUSCS | Lower Uterine Segment Caesarean Section |
| LVF | Left Ventricular Failure |
| MAC | Minimum Alveolar Concentration |
| MAP | Mean arterial pressure |
| MCP | Metacarpophalangeal |
| MH | Malignant hyperthermia (Pyrexia) |
| MI | Myocardial infarction |
| MMR | Measles, Mumps & Rubella |
| MMV | Mandatory Minute Volume |
| MOP | Mean Arterial Pressure |
| MRI | Magnetic resonance imaging |
| MS | Multiple Sclerosis |
| MSU | Mid Stream Urine |
| MTP | Metarsophalangeal |
| MUA | Manipulation under anaesthetic |
| MV | Minute volume |
| $N_2O$ | Nitrous oxide |
| NAASP | National Association of Assistants in Surgical Practice |
| NaCl | Sodium chloride |
| NATN | National Association of Theatre Nurses |
| NBM | Nil by mouth |
| NFR | Not for resuscitation |
| NGT | Nasogastric tube |
| NMC | Nursing & Midwifery Council |
| NSAID | Non-steroidal anti-inflammatory drug |
| $O_2$ | Oxygen |
| OE | On Examination |
| OGD | Oesophago Gastro Duodenoscopy |
| OPD | Out Patient Department |
| ORIF | Open reduction internal fixation |
| PA | Pulmonary Artery |
| PACU | Post Anaesthetic Care Unit |
| PALS | Paediatric Advanced Life Support |
| PAW | Pulmonary Artery Wedge |
| PCA | Patient controlled analgesia |
| PCV | Packed Cell Volume |
| PCWP | Pulmonary Capillary Wedge Pressure |
| PE | Pulmonary embolus |

| | |
|---|---|
| PEEP | Positive end expiratory pressure |
| PEG | Percutaneous Endoscopic Gastrostomy |
| PERLA | Pupils equal and reacting to light and accommodation |
| PIP | Proximal interphalangeal joint |
| PM | Postmortem |
| PMH | Past Medical History |
| PNS | Postnasal space |
| PONV | Post-operative nausea and vomiting |
| POP | Plaster of Paris |
| PP | Placenta Praevia |
| PPE | Personal Protective Equipment |
| PPF | Plasma Protein Fraction |
| PPH | Post Partum Haemorrhage |
| PPM | Parts per million |
| PR | Per rectum |
| PRN | Pro re nata (when required) |
| PT | Prothrombin time |
| PTSD | Post-traumatic stress disorder |
| PU | Peptic Ulcer |
| PV | Per vagina |
| QA | Quality Assurance |
| QDS | Four times a day |
| RCN | Royal College of Nursing |
| REM | Rapid Eye Movement |
| RIDDOR | Reporting of Injuries, Diseases and Dangerous Occurrences Regulations |
| RIF | Right iliac fossa |
| RIH | Right inguinal hernia |
| RR | Respiratory rate |
| RSI | Repetitive Strain Injury |
| RTA | Road Traffic Accident |
| SA | Surgical Assistant |
| SADS | Seasonal Affective Disorder Syndrome |
| SCBU | Special Care Baby Unit |
| SI | Systems International |
| SIMV | Synchronised intermittent mandatory ventilation |
| SMR | Submucous resection |
| SP | Surgical Practitioner |
| STD | Sexually Transmitted Disease |
| SVT | Supraventricular tachycardia |
| T&As | Tonsils and adenoids |
| TAH | Total abdominal hysterectomy |
| TB | Tuberculosis |
| TCRE | Trans Cervical Resection of Endometrium |
| Td | Tetanus, diphtheria |

**Operating Department Practice A–Z**

| | |
|---|---|
| TDS | Three times a day |
| TENS | Transcutaneous electrical nerve simulation |
| THR | Total hip replacement |
| TIA | Transient ischaemic attack |
| TIVA | Total intravenous anaesthesia |
| TKR | Total knee replacement |
| TL | Tubal Ligation |
| To4 | Train of Four |
| TOP | Termination of Pregnancy |
| TPN | Total parenteral nutrition |
| TPR | Temperature pulse and respiration |
| TSSU | Theatre Sterile Services Unit |
| TTO | To take out |
| TURBN | Trans Urethral Resection of Bladder Neck |
| TURP | Transurethral resection of prostate |
| TURT | Transurethral resection of tumour |
| TV | Tidal volume |
| TVH | Total Vaginal Hysterectomy |
| U&Es | Urea and Electrolyte |
| URTI | Upper respiratory tract infection |
| USS | Ultra Sound Scan |
| UTI | Urinary tract infection |
| UV | Ultraviolet |
| Var | Varicella (chicken pox) |
| VC | Vital Capacity |
| VF | Ventricular fibrillation |
| VT | Ventricular tachycardia |
| VTOP | Vacuum Termination of Pregnancy |
| VVs | Varicose veins |
| WBC | White Blood Count |
| WHO | World Health Organisation |
| Wt | Weight |
| YOB | Year of Birth |
| ↓ | Decreased or lowered |
| ↑ | Increase or raised |
| # | Fracture |

**Abdomen**   *Quick Reference:* The area of the body between the chest and the pelvis.

*Advanced Reference:* The abdomen is separated from the chest by the *diaphragm*. The contents of the abdomen include the *stomach, small intestine, colon, rectum, liver, spleen, pancreas, kidneys, appendix, gall bladder* and *urinary bladder*.

**Abdominal aortic aneurysm**   *Quick Reference:* (an-your-ism) A ballooning or dilatation of the aorta in the abdominal region.

*Advanced Reference:* The aneurysm weakens the wall of the aorta and can result in the aorta rupturing with potentially fatal consequences. As the diameter of the aorta increases, the chances of rupture also increase. Men, usually over 60, are five times more likely than women to suffer this type of aneurysm. Also referred to as *triple A* (*AAA*).

**Abdominal hysterectomy**   *Quick Reference:* (hist-er-ec-tommy) The surgical removal of the uterus through an incision in the abdominal wall.

*Advanced Reference:* The procedure involves a number of approaches depending on severity and/or spread, i.e. total, sub-total, *pan, Wertheims*.

**Abdomino-perineal**   *Quick Reference:* Pertaining to the abdomen and perineum.

*Advanced Reference:* Includes the pelvic area, the female vulva and anus, and the male anus and scrotum. An abdomino-perineal resection procedure involves excision of the lower colon, rectum and anus.

**Abduction**   *Quick Reference:* The opposite of *adduction*.

*Advanced Reference:* The movement of a limb away from the midline of the body. Abduction of the legs is, therefore, to spread the legs (outwards).

**Aberrant**   *Quick Reference:* Pertaining to a wandering from the usual or expected pathway.

*Advanced Reference:* Can be applied to the heart when the electrical system does not follow the usual conduction route.

**Ablation**   *Quick Reference:* Removal or destruction.

*Advanced Reference:* The removal or destruction of body tissue, usually by surgical means. The most common being ablation of the uterus.

**Abortion**   *Quick Reference:* The loss of a pregnancy.

*Advanced Reference:* The premature exit of the products of conception (the foetus, foetal membranes and placenta) from the uterus. The term does not refer to why or how the pregnancy was lost. A spontaneous abortion is commonly called 'a miscarriage'.

**Abruption**   *Quick Reference:* A sudden breaking off or tearing apart.

*Advanced Reference:* Placental abruption indicates the separation of the placenta from the normal position of the uterus during pregnancy and usually refers to the period after 20 weeks. Results in severe *haemorrhage*.

**Abscess**   *Quick Reference:* (ab-ses) A collection of pus as the result of infection.

*Advanced Reference:* An abscess forms as the result of infection. The area of infection becomes isolated from the healthy tissue and in time the dead white blood cells, bacteria and fluid form pus.

**Acetabulum**   *Quick Reference:* (as-e-tab-u-lum) A cup-shaped cavity on the outer side of the femur.

*Advanced Reference*: Indicates the socket of the hip joint in which the head of the femur moves (articulates).

**Acetylcholine**   *Quick Reference:* (a-seat-al-coal-een) A neurotransmitter.

*Advanced Reference:* Involved in the transmission of nervous impulses between nerve endings and the muscles and within the parasympathetic nervous system. Is broken down normally by *cholinesterase*. Muscle relaxant drugs act by competing with acetylcholine at the neuromuscular junction.

**Achilles tendon**   *Quick Reference:* (a-kill-ease) Tendon which runs from the calf muscle to the heel.

*Advanced Reference:* The achilles is responsible for drawing the foot downwards, hinging at the ankle joint. Is a weak point in certain sports and can rupture during activity and consequently requires surgical repair.

**Acid–base balance**   *Quick Reference:* Indicates a balance in the production and secretion of acids and bases.

*Advanced Reference:* A balance provides a stable concentration of hydrogen ions in the body.

**Acidosis**   *Quick Reference:* Alteration of the *acid–alkali* balance of blood and tissue fluid towards acidity.

*Advanced Reference:* In health, the slight alkalinity is held constant by the balance of dissolved *carbon dioxide* ($CO_2$, acid) and *sodium bicarbonate* (alkali). Can be of metabolic or respiratory nature. A person suffering acidosis is said to be an acidotic.

**Acquired immunity**   *Quick Reference:* Form of immunity that is not innate.
*Advanced Reference:* Obtained during life and may be naturally or artificially acquired or passively induced.

**ACTH**   *Quick Reference:* Abbreviation for adrenocorticotrophic hormone.
*Advanced Reference:* A secretion of the *pituitary* gland which has the function of stimulating the cortex of the adrenal gland to secrete cortisone.

**Actrapid**   *Quick Reference:* Proprietary quick acting preparation of insulin.
*Advanced Reference:* Used to treat patients with diabetes mellitus.

**Acute abdomen**   *Quick Reference:* The sudden severe onset of abdominal pain.
*Advanced Reference:* Referred to a potential medical emergency, indicating a potentially major problem with one of the abdominal organs, e.g. a ruptured appendix, inflamed gall bladder or ruptured spleen.

**Adams apple**   *Quick Reference:* Thyroid cartilage.
*Advanced Reference:* Positioned at the anterior of the larynx and showing as a protrusion at the front of the neck, more prominent in men than women due to anatomical positioning.

**Adduction**   *Quick Reference:* The opposite of *abduction*.
*Advanced Reference:* The movement of a limb into (towards) the midline of the body. Adduction would bring the legs together.

**Adenosine**   *Quick Reference:* Endogenous nucleoside.
*Advanced Reference:* Drug used to treat supraventricular *tachycardia* (SVT) and ascertain the nature of other tachycardias.

**ADH**   *Quick Reference:* Antidiuretic hormone. Also known as *vasopressin*.
*Advanced Reference:* Released by the pituitary gland and promotes water re-absorption in the kidney tubules. Those suffering diabetes insipidus lack ADH. Is now used in the form of vasopressin as an alternative to *adrenaline* during cardiopulmonary resuscitation (*CPR*).

**Adhesion**   *Quick Reference:* The joining or sticking together of two surfaces that are normally separated.
*Advanced Reference:* Adhesions can occur as a result of *inflammation* which causes fibrous tissue to form. For example, peritonitis can cause adhesions which may then lead to intestinal obstruction. Also may be due to previous surgery.

**Adrenaline (Epinephrine)**   *Quick Reference:* A hormone secreted by the medulla of the adrenal gland.

*Advanced Reference:* Also known by its drug name 'epinephrine'. Stimulates the heart action, raises blood pressure (BP), releases glucose and increases its metabolism, increases muscular blood circulation, relaxes air passages, etc. Hence, it is useful in situations of shock and resuscitation.

**Advocate** *Quick Reference:* One who acts on the behalf of others.
*Advanced Reference:* Anyone who acts in support of the patient, especially if they are unable to speak or act for themselves.

**Afferent** *Quick Reference:* Towards the centre.
*Advanced Reference:* Afferent vessels and structures run throughout the body, i.e. the small arterioles entering the *glomerulus* of the kidney, the sensory nerve fibres that convey impulses from the periphery to the brain, and lymphatic vessels that lead from the tissues to a *lymph* gland.

**Agar** *Quick Reference:* Culture medium.
*Advanced Reference:* Composed of seaweed with a broth or blood added as a nutrient. Resists the digestive action of bacteria and therefore used as a medium on which cultures can be grown. Not all micro-organisms will grow in such a way outside of the body. Viruses require living tissue to survive.

**Agglutination** *Quick Reference:* The coming together of small particles in a solution to form clumps.
*Advanced Reference:* In blood, it is brought about by the action of antibodies on antigens carried by red blood cells or bacteria and is therefore utilised to identify blood groups during cross-matching (X-matching).

**Aggregate** *Quick Reference:* To gather together.
*Advanced Reference:* Indicates the total of a group of substances or components making up a mass or complex.

**Agonal** *Quick Reference:* Pertaining to death and dying.
*Advanced Reference:* An agonal electrocardiography (ECG) rhythm indicates a trace that displays a dying heart.

**Agonist** *Quick Reference:* Opposite to *antagonist*; to act against or has opposing action.
*Advanced Reference:* The term applied to the action of drugs, i.e. an antagonist is given to block the effect of an agonist. Also used with reference to the action of muscles.

**Alberti** *Quick Reference:* A diabetic protocol.
*Advanced Reference:* Involves 10 units of *actrapid* insulin and 10 mmol of *potassium chloride* added to 500 ml 10% *dextrose* and infused over 4 hours. A fail-safe system means that variations in infusion rate cannot produce an imbalance of glucose and insulin and so hypokalaemia.

**Albumin**   *Quick Reference:* A plasma protein.
*Advanced Reference:* Also an intravenous (IV) *plasma expander* (**HAS**, human albumin solution).

**Aldasorber**   *Quick Reference:* Passive scavenging system.
*Advanced Reference:* Prior to establishment of active scavenging systems, the Aldasorber passive system was used in many centres. Involves a scavenging valve and tubing which is connected to a small container of activated charcoal which absorbs *halothane* from expired gases. Containers had to be disposed of when they reached a stated weight.

**Aldehyde**   *Quick Reference:* Colourless volatile fluid with suffocating smell.
*Advanced Reference:* Obtained by oxidation of alcohol, acetaldehyde. Seen in the theatres as formaldehyde and *gluteraldehyde*.

**Aldosterone**   *Quick Reference:* Hormone released by the renal cortex.
*Advanced Reference:* Responsible for the regulation of sodium levels in the body by re-absorption in the kidney. In order to balance electrolytes, this hormone also plays a part in potassium excretion.

**Alfentanil**   *Quick Reference:* Narcotic analgesia, e.g. Rapifen.
*Advanced Reference:* Used for short surgical procedures and outpatients/day-case surgery. Also used as infusion during prolonged procedures.

**Alimentary**   *Quick Reference:* Refers to the alimentary canal or digestive tract.
*Advanced Reference:* The alimentary tract is composed of the mouth, pharynx, oesophagus, stomach and intestine.

**Alkali**   *Quick Reference:* Substance which neutralises acid to produce a salt.
*Advanced Reference:* Most common alkalis are oxides, hydroxides or carbonates and bicarbonates. Examples are sodium bicarbonate, calcium carbonate, magnesium carbonate, magnesium trisilicate and aluminium hydroxide. Alkalis turn red litmus blue. Alkalosis is an increase in body alkali reserve, in other words a high pH. Due to several causes, such as acid loss through vomiting, etc., or in the event of an alkali (bicarbonate) intake.

**Alkaloids**   *Quick Reference:* Large group of alkaline substances found in plants.
*Advanced Reference:* Widely used in medicine. Common examples are *atropine*, *cocaine*, *caffeine*, *morphine*, *codeine*, *quinine* and *nicotine*. All have names ending in 'ine'.

**Alkalosis**   *Quick Reference:* Condition in which the body's pH increases.
*Advanced Reference:* An acid–base imbalance in which there is a decrease in the hydrogen ion concentration and an increase in the pH.

Common causes are carbonic acid deficit or an excessive amount of bicarbonate. May be classified as respiratory or metabolic.

**Allergy**  *Quick Reference:* Hypersensitivity to various substances (allergens), e.g. drugs, foods and insect bites.
 *Advanced Reference:* It is due to an antigen–antibody reaction. Hay fever and asthma are examples of an allergic reaction.

**Alloferin**  *Quick Reference:* Proprietary non-depolarising muscle relaxant.
 *Advanced Reference:* Synthetic non-depolarising muscle relaxant with a duration of 20–30 min; is a preparation of alcuronium chloride.

**Allograft**  *Quick Reference:* Type of graft or transplant.
 *Advanced Reference:* A graft or *transplant* between different species.

**Alloy**  *Quick Reference:* To combine metals.
 *Advanced Reference:* A mixture of two or more metals or substances with metallic properties. Those with a medical application include amalgam (mercury and silver) used in tooth fillings, also many are used in the manufacture of joint prosthesis.

**Ambu bag**  *Quick Reference:* Trade name of a resuscitation device.
 *Advanced Reference:* Used as a general term to indicate airway management devices with a one-way valve used in resuscitation. It is now a general design of devices more generally referred to as bagvalve mask (*BVM*).

**Aminophylline**  *Quick Reference:* (amin-off-i-lean) Bronchodilator drug.
 *Advanced Reference:* Used to treat moderate forms of asthma and pulmonary oedema.

**Amiodarone**  *Quick Reference:* Anti-arrhythmic drug, e.g. cordarone.
 *Advanced Reference:* Used to treat resistant *SVT*. Now available instead of an alternative to *lignocaine* during cardiac resuscitation.

**Ammonia**  *Quick Reference:* A colourless pungent gas.
 *Advanced Reference:* Produced by the decomposition of nitrogenous organic matter.

**Amnesia**  *Quick Reference:* Loss of memory.
 *Advanced Reference:* Caused usually by injury or emotional trauma.

**Amniotic**  *Quick Reference:* Refers to amniotic fluid inside the pregnant uterus.
 *Advanced Reference:* The amnion is a membranous bag containing the amniotic fluid, a watery liquid in which the baby floats until birth. Amniocentesis is the withdrawal of amniotic fluid from the uterus through the abdominal wall and used for diagnosis of chromosome disorders in the foetus.

**Amoxil**   *Quick Reference:* Proprietary antibiotic.

*Advanced Reference:* Used in the treatment of systemic bacterial infections and those of the upper respiratory tract, ear, nose and throat, and urogenital tract. Is a preparation of a broad-spectrum penicillin, amoxycillin.

**Amp**   *Quick Reference:* Ampere.

*Advanced Reference:* Unit of measurement of amount of electrical current.

**Ampicillin**   *Quick Reference:* Broad-spectrum antibiotic.

*Advanced Reference:* Similar in effect to tetracyclines. Used in the treatment of urogenital tract, upper respiratory and ear infections. Many bacteria now have become resistant to this drug.

**Amplitude**   *Quick Reference:* Width or breadth of range.

*Advanced Reference:* Maximum extent of vibration or oscillation from a position of equilibrium. The amplitude is the height/strength of an ECG signal.

**Ampoule**   *Quick Reference:* Small glass or plastic container or vial.

*Advanced Reference:* Designed to contain a single dose of a drug or solution, as opposed to a multi-dose vial.

**Anaemia**   *Quick Reference:* (an-eem-ea) Condition in which there is an insufficient amount of oxygen-carrying capacity in the blood.

*Advanced Reference:* Various forms exist, e.g. iron-deficiency anaemia, haemolytic anaemia, pernicious anaemia, thalassaemia, *sickle-cell anaemia.*

**Anaerobic**   *Quick Reference:* (an-air-obic) Living without oxygen.

*Advanced Reference:* An anaerobic micro-organism is one that can survive in the absence of oxygen, e.g. those that cause tetanus and gas gangrene or are found in wounds and body cavities which are either free of or low in oxygen, i.e. the bowel.

**Anaesthesia**   *Quick Reference:* Literally means without feeling.

*Advanced Reference:* Term which indicates both general and local anaesthesia (GA and LA, respectively) and also used interchangeably with *analgesia.* Commonly understood to indicate, being put to sleep in order to undergo surgery.

**Analgesia**   *Quick Reference:* Indicates without pain.

*Advanced Reference:* Often used interchangeably with *anaesthesia,* which actually indicates without feeling. Primarily involves drugs and medicines given for pain relief. Referred to as analgesics.

**Anaphylaxis**   *Quick Reference:* (ana-falax-is) A category of shock caused by a second exposure to a foreign protein (allergen), a substance capable of causing an allergy.

*Advanced Reference:* The initial exposure to the allergen has made the person abnormally sensitive and leads to an immediate reaction. Signs and symptoms are as for shock or allergic reaction, i.e. skin rash (***urticaria***), tachycardia, vasodilatation, hypotension, sweating, ***dyspnoea***, bronchial swelling, etc. Symptoms are mainly due to histamine release. *Anaphylactoid* reaction is different from anaphylaxis in that it is not immune related but more a reaction to a substance which causes histamine release.

**Anastomosis** *Quick Reference:* Artificial opening between two hollow structures.

*Advanced Reference:* In surgery, anastomosis is the joining of two ends of a structure usually following resection, i.e. between the two cut-ends of stomach or intestine when part has been removed. Also when joining blood vessel ends or vessel end to a graft.

**Anatomical snuffbox** *Quick Reference:* Small cup-like depression on the back of the hand near the wrist.

*Advanced Reference:* Formed by tendons reaching towards the thumb and index finger.

**Aneroid** *Quick Reference:* Indicates absence of fluid or not containing water.

*Advanced Reference:* Used to describe a device that is in contrast to one that utilises or contains fluid, e.g. an aneroid sphygmomanometer, which contains no mercury.

**Aneurysm** *Quick Reference:* (an-your-ism) Local dilatation of an artery sometimes forming a sac.

*Advanced Reference:* May be congenital due to inflammation or caused by trauma. The pressure of blood causes it to distend and become prone to rupture. Common sites are the abdominal aorta, carotid artery in the neck. There are a number of variations including, dissecting aneurysm in which a tear occurs in the lining and blood makes its way between the layers of the vessel forcing them apart, also saccular aneurysm which involves only a part of the arterial circumference dilating. Treatment for all usually involves surgery for repair, or more likely, grafting.

**Angina pectoris** *Quick Reference*: Severe chest pain.

*Advanced Reference:* Pectoris indicates the region of the pectoral muscle of the chest. The pain is due to occlusion or spasm of the main arteries (coronary) supplying the heart, leading to lack of oxygen to the heart muscle itself. Hence, demand outstrips supply. Relieved by vasodilator drugs, i.e. glyceryl trinitrate (nitroglycerine, GTN) which can be administered by tablet or absorbed from under the tongue (sublingual).

**Angiography** *Quick Reference:* X-ray of the cerebral vascular tree.

*Advanced Reference:* Involves imaging following the injection of a radio-opaque medium into a main neck artery.

**Angioplasty**   *Quick Reference:* Dilatation of a blocked blood vessel.
*Advanced Reference:* Balloon angioplasty usually involves dilatation of a blocked or constricted artery.

**Anion**   *Quick Reference:* A negatively charged ion.
*Advanced Reference:* An ion in an electrolysed solution that migrates to the anode. The anode being the positive pole and cathode the negative.

**Ankylosing spondylitis**   *Quick Reference:* (ankal-osing) Type of *arthritis* causing deformity and stiffness.
*Advanced Reference:* The resultant inflammation affects the joint capsules, attached *ligaments* and *tendons*. If present in the area of the neck and spine can cause severe deformity (*kyphosis*) which may lead to airway management problems during anaesthesia.

**Anorexia**   *Quick Reference:* Dietary disease also known as the slimmer's disease.
*Advanced Reference:* Correct term is anorexia nervosa. Symptoms include patients refusing to eat or eat only under protest, they may also vomit to get rid of food. Leads to nutritional deficiency and hormonal upset. Occurs mainly in females between the ages of 14 and 17.

**Antacid**   *Quick Reference:* Substance used to neutralise stomach acid.
*Advanced Reference*: In relation to the *peri-operative* period, antacids are used for patients who are at risk of *regurgitation* possibly due to *hiatus hernia*, gastro-oesophageal reflux, etc., given pre-operatively. Sodium citrate is common for *Caesarean section* patients. *Sodium bicarbonate*, aluminium hydroxide, *magnesium* trisilicate are further examples of antacids.

**Antagonist**   *Quick Reference:* An opposite or opposing action to another.
*Advanced Reference:* Examples would be the muscles, biceps and triceps; one relaxes to allow the other to contract. With reference to drugs, indicates one which blocks or reverses the action of another.

**Antecubital fossa**   *Quick Reference:* Inside area of the elbow.
*Advanced Reference:* Area on the inside of the elbow where access for *cannulation* is made via the *basilic* and *cephalic* veins (ante: before; cubitus: forearm; fossa: depression or pit).

**Anteflexion**   *Quick Reference:* Bending forward.
*Advanced Reference:* The uterus is a prime example of an organ that bends forward.

**Antepartum**   *Quick Reference:* Before childbirth.
*Advanced Reference:* Actually indicates the 3-month period prior to giving birth. An antepartum haemorrhage is bleeding from the uterus before delivery caused by the dislodged placenta lying below the baby.

**Anterior**   *Quick Reference:* Indicates front.

*Advanced Reference:* Opposite to *posterior*. Foremost, front surface of, etc. *Ventral* is also used to indicate the front surface of the body.

**Anteverted**   *Quick Reference:* Tilted forward.

*Advanced Reference:* Indicates the forward tilting of an organ, as with the uterus which has a normal position of being tilted slightly forward.

**Anti-arrhythmic**   *Quick Reference:* (a-rith-mic) Range of drugs used to regulate the heartbeat.

*Advanced Reference:* As there are a number of ways in which the heartbeat can become irregular, the range of drugs to treat this is also broad. Irregularities include atrial and ventricular tachycardia, atrial flutter and fibrillation as well as the changes that may follow a heart attack. Common anti-arrhythmic drugs include: *digoxin*, *verapamil*, *lignocaine* and *amiodarone*.

**Antibacterials**   *Quick Reference:* Drugs and substances that destroy bacteria but may have less effect on other micro-organisms.

*Advanced Reference:* The major group involved is antibiotics, although sulphonamides are sometimes categorised as such, they have specific uses or are administered in combination with antibiotics especially where resistant strains or sensitivity are involved.

**Antibiotic**   *Quick Reference:* A class of drugs used to treat infections.

*Advanced Reference:* Collective name for a class of substances produced by living organisms which are capable of destroying or hindering growth of pathogenic organisms. The term is also used to cover similar synthetic compounds which have the same function. The action of one type of microbe opposing the growth of another (antagonism) is termed antibiosis.

**Antibody**   *Quick Reference:* Against (the body).

*Advanced Reference:* Specific substances produced in the blood as a reaction to an *antigen* (foreign substance).

**Anticancer**   *Quick Reference:* The drugs involved here are mostly *cytotoxics*.

*Advanced Reference:* They work by interfering with cell replication or production and so preventing growth of new tissue. Inevitably, this means that normal cell production is also affected and therefore may produce some severe side effects.

**Anticholinergic**   *Quick Reference:* Drugs that inhibit the action, release or production of the substance acetylcholine.

*Advanced Reference:* Acetylcholine plays an important part in the nervous system, tending to relax smooth muscle. Atropine is an example of an anticholinergic drug.

**Anticholinesterases**   *Quick Reference:* (anti-cole-in-est-erase) Agents which inhibit cholinesterases.

*Advanced Reference:* These drugs increase the concentration of acetyl-choline at the neuromuscular junction and as this substance causes depolarisation they tend to have a depolarising action.

**Antidote**   *Quick Reference:* Substance given to counteract or neutralise the effects of, e.g. a poison.
*Advanced Reference*: Example would be an alkali neutralising an acid. Commonly used in reference to snake venom.

**Anti-emetic**   *Quick Reference:* Drug given to prevent vomiting.
*Advanced Reference:* This group of drugs work by either directly affect-ing the vomit centre in the brain or by stimulating gastrointestinal emptying.

**Antigen**   *Quick Reference:* A substance treated as alien to the body's natural components.
*Advanced Reference:* Any substance which invokes the action of an *antibody.*

**Antihistamine**   *Quick Reference:* Drug which counteracts the effects of *histamine.*
*Advanced Reference:* Antihistamines work by blocking the receptors for histamine. Used in the treatment of drug allergies, allergic and itching rashes and urticaria.

**Antiseptic**   *Quick Reference:* Substance that destroys or arrests the devel-opment of bacteria.
*Advanced Reference:* Used interchangeably but wrongly with disinfec-tant. One difference being that antiseptics can be safely applied to the body whereas disinfectants generally cannot. Antiseptics are used primarily to prevent infection.

**Antisialagogues**   *Quick Reference:* (anti-sial-og-us) Drying of salivary secretions.
*Advanced Reference:* Drugs in this group, *atropine* being most com-mon, have the action of drying both salivary and bronchial secretions. Useful in *premedication.*

**Antrum**   *Quick Reference:* A cavity or chamber.
*Advanced Reference:* One that is nearly closed and usually surrounded by bone.

**Apache**   *Quick Reference:* **A**cute **P**hysiology **A**nd **C**hronic **H**ealth **E**valuation.
*Advanced Reference:* A scoring system of severity of illness in intensive therapy unit (*ITU*) patients.

**Aperture**   *Quick Reference:* An opening or hole.
*Advanced Reference:* May be present in an object or anatomical structure.

**Apex**   *Quick Reference:* The summit, top or peak of anything cone shaped. As with the summit (apex) of a mountain.

A

*Advanced Reference:* Used with reference to the apex beat of the heart, located or felt at the level of the fifth left intercostals space in the mid-clavicular line.

**Apgar scale**   *Quick Reference:* A scoring system used to assess the new born.

*Advanced Reference:* Involves assessment of pulse/heart rate, respiratory effort, muscle tone, grimace/irritability and colour. Each is awarded a value $(0, 1, 2)$ and total score indicates condition, maximum 10, below 9 requires attention and less than 6 indicates infant needs resuscitation. Taken at 1- and 5-minute intervals after birth.

**Apnoea**   *Quick Reference:* Cessation of breathing.

*Advanced Reference:* Due to a number of factors. Commonly involves a drop in the necessary $CO_2$ tension in the blood in order to stimulate the respiratory centre.

**Appendicectomy**   *Quick Reference:* (appen-dis-ectomy) Surgical removal of the appendix.

*Advanced Reference:* Identification of the *appendix* at the *ileo-caecal* junction, i.e. the distal aspects of the *ileum* and the **proximal** aspects of ascending **colon**. Removal of the appendix utilising a purse-string suture. The McBurney point is the name given to the surgical incision site.

**Apronectomy**   *Quick Reference:* A plastic surgery procedure carried out for obesity.

*Advanced Reference:* Involves removal of an apron of skin and underlying fat from the abdomino-pelvic region, mainly for cosmetic indications.

**Aramine**   *Quick Reference:* Vasoconstrictor drug.

*Advanced Reference:* Proprietary form of metaraminol. Used to raise BP or in conditions of severe shock. During anaesthesia it is used as either injection or infusion.

**ARDS**   *Quick Reference:* Adult respiratory distress syndrome.

*Advanced Reference:* Serious disease of the lungs, with a high mortality rate. A form of respiratory failure due to a number of causes. Predisposing factors include aspiration of gastric contents, sepsis, fluid overload and lung contusion.

**Arm board**   *Quick Reference:* Piece of equipment used to support and position the patient's arm(s) during surgery.

*Advanced Reference:* Positioned from the side of the operating table at shoulder level as a support when the arm is at an angle to the table. Intended to give access to the arm/hand for IV access and BP readings, etc., as well as keeping the arm clear of the surgical site. There are a number of inherent hazards involved in the use of arm boards: (1) The angle of the board must not exceed 90° as this could cause brachial plexus injury. (2) The board can drop below the table level causing a drag on the shoulder joint and associated nerves. (3) As some are made of metal, earthing of the patient's skin is possible if unprotected. (4) There are opposing views over whether the arm/hand should lie palm up or palm down and any benefits of the patient's head facing towards the arm out on a board in order to reduce anatomical stress. Also, having both arms out simultaneously creates the potential for injury if necessary precautions are not identified. There are designs of arm board available for both attaching to the table and sliding under the table mattress.

**Arm support** *Quick Reference:* Device for securing the patient's arms at their side during surgery.

*Advanced Reference:* Numerous models are available but all are a variation on an L-shaped plastic design. Intended to fit under the table mattress with the upper section supporting the arms, whether positioned at the patient's side or folded across the chest. If wrongly applied, can cause pressure damage to the arm itself and the ulnar nerve at the elbow as well as skin damage if placed directly under the patient and not the mattress.

**Arrhythmia** *Quick Reference:* (a-rith-mea) Any irregularity in the rhythm of the heartbeat.

*Advanced Reference:* Actually indicates no rhythm so is an inaccurate term. **Dysrhythmia** is more accurate. Drugs used to treat arrhythmias are known as anti-arrhythmics. **Lignocaine** and *amiodarone* are commonly used in the treatment of tachy-arrhythmias.

**Artefact** *Quick Reference:* Artificially made.

*Advanced Reference:* False signals, etc. Interference in radiology, ECG trace, etc.

**Arteriosclerosis** *Quick Reference:* Hardening of the arteries.

*Advanced Reference:* Loss of elasticity of the arterial walls due to thickening and calcification. Leads to raised BP.

**Artery forceps** *Quick Reference:* An instrument for holding *'bleeders'* securely.

*Advanced Reference:* All artery forceps have serrated jaws designed to hold bleeding vessels securely. Some have sharp teeth at the ends of their jaws which provide a stronger grip on tough tissues. Artery forceps come in many sizes and shapes, with some of the most common being Mosquito, Halstead, Spencer Wells, Kelly and Kocher. Known as 'clamp'.

**Arthritis** *Quick Reference:* Inflammation of a joint.

*Advanced Reference:* Term applied to many types of joint disease, although not always accurately. A degenerative condition in which the restriction of movement is a prominent factor. The three common types of arthritis are: rheumatoid, osteo and gout.

**Arthroplasty** *Quick Reference:* Replacement of a joint with an artificial device.

*Advanced Reference:* The joint being replaced by a prosthesis. Arthro meaning joint and plasty indicating a moulding, i.e. total knee *arthroplasty*, where the distal end of the femur and the head of the tibia both replaced with a plastic prosthesis.

**Articular**   *Quick Reference:* Pertaining to a joint.
*Advanced Reference:* Indicates a joint or the movement of joints.

**Arytenoid**   *Quick Reference:* (aret-noid) cartilages (2) to the larynx.
*Advanced Reference:* Their function is to adjust the tension of the vocal cords to which they are attached.

**ASA**   *Quick Reference:* American Society of Anaesthetists.
*Advanced Reference:* Refers to the criteria laid down by the ASA which involves a patient's pre-operative assessment, and classification which utilises a scale of 1–5 ranging from healthy to moribund which also includes emergency status.

**Asbestos**   *Quick Reference:* Combination of minerals, i.e. magnesium silicate. At one time commonly used in the building trade in the structures or as insulation.
*Advanced Reference:* Inhalation of the dust can lead to pulmonary fibrosis and cancer. Asbestosis, accumulation in the bronchioles. One type of asbestos is responsible for *mesothelioma*. Now tightly controlled under Health and Safety Law.

**Ascites**   *Quick Reference:* (a-site-ees) Accumulation of fluid in the peritoneum.
*Advanced Reference:* Leads to swelling in such conditions as heart, kidney and liver disease which can bring about *exudation* from the blood vessels. *Paracentesis* is a procedure performed to draw off the fluid with a needle entering through the abdominal wall.

**Asepsis**   *Quick Reference:* Absence of any living organism.
*Advanced Reference:* Term often used interchangeably but wrongly with sterile. In relation to theatres, indicates an area intended to be free of micro-organisms by the use of antiseptics, barriers, washing techniques, etc.

**Asthma**   *Quick Reference:* (as-th-ma) respiratory disease which produces attacks of breathing difficulty.
*Advanced Reference:* Asthma attacks produce difficulty in expiration, due to hypersensitivity to foreign substances. Involves narrowing of the bronchi, this reverses either spontaneously or in response to medication.

**Astringent**   *Quick Reference:* Agent that causes contraction of tissues upon application.
*Advanced Reference:* Used locally on skin, etc. Stops capillary bleeding, loosens secretions, etc.

**Asymmetrical**   *Quick Reference:* Unequal in size or shape.
*Advanced Reference:* Different in placement and arrangement (about an axis).

**Asystole**   *Quick Reference:* (a-sis-toe-lee) Absence of the heartbeat.
*Advanced Reference:* Confirmed when no ventricular activity is seen on the Electrocardiograph (ECG) trace.

**Ataxia**   *Quick Reference:* Impaired ability to co-ordinate movement.
*Advanced Reference:* Involves posture imbalance. Causing someone to stagger, etc.

**Atelectasis**   *Quick Reference:* (atel-ac-tesis) Incomplete expansion of the lung.
*Advanced Reference:* A term that may cover a number of causes and effects in both infants and adults. Also described as collapse of the lung.

**Atenolol**   *Quick Reference:* A **beta-blocker** drug.
*Advanced Reference:* Used to reduce the heart rate and force of contraction.

**Atheroma**   *Quick Reference:* Fatty deposit.
*Advanced Reference:* Causes thickening of arterial walls and blockages composed of fatty substances such as cholesterol.

**Atherosclerosis**   *Quick Reference:* Disease of the walls of arteries.
*Advanced Reference:* The walls of the arteries become thickened, stiff and swollen following the laying down of atheromatous deposits.

**Atracurium**   *Quick Reference:* Tracrium. A skeletal muscle relaxant.
*Advanced Reference:* Non-depolarising muscle relaxant with a duration of 20–25 min; often the drug of choice in renal and hepatic impairment. Undergoes spontaneous degradation due to a process known as Hoffman elimination and therefore spontaneous reversal.

**Atropine**   *Quick Reference:* An anticholinergic.
*Advanced Reference:* Obtained from belladonna (deadly nightshade). Used in combination with neostigmine during reversal of non-depolarising muscle relaxants. Commonly used in combination with tranquillisers and narcotics as a premedication has the effects of drying salivary secretions and is an antispasmodic. Used to dilate the pupil of the eye for ophthalmic surgery.

**Auditory**   *Quick Reference:* Pertaining to the sense of hearing.
*Advanced Reference:* Audiology is the science of dealing with hearing and audiometry is the measurement of the power of hearing.

**Augmentin**   *Quick Reference:* Commonly used antibiotic.
*Advanced Reference:* Proprietary preparation of the penicillin-like antibiotic amoxycillin combined with an extending agent, clavulanic acid, which extends the action and power of amoxycillin.

**Ausculation**   *Quick Reference:* (os-cue-lation) Method of examining the body by listening.
*Advanced Reference:* Mostly applies to the chest and heart when being examined with a **stethoscope**.

A

**Autoclave**   *Quick Reference:* A machine for sterilising equipment.

*Advanced Reference:* The autoclave is a machine that uses steam and pressure to sterilise surgical instruments. It will destroy most *micro-organisms*, such as human immunodeficiency virus (*HIV*) but will not kill Creutzfeldt–Jakob disease (*CJD*).

**Autograft**   *Quick Reference:* Graft from one part of the same body to another. Auto indicates self.

*Advanced Reference:* A graft where the donor is also the *recipient*, e.g. skin graft.

**Autonomic nervous system**   *Quick Reference:* Regulates body functions other than voluntary movement and conscious sensation.

*Advanced Reference:* Composed of the sympathetic and parasympathetic nervous systems whose actions are generally opposed, e.g. the sympathetic accelerates the heart and the parasympathetic slows down, while e.g. on the intestine they function the other way round.

**AV fistula**   *Quick Reference:* Fistula indicates a false or abnormal passage connecting one structure with another.

*Advanced Reference:* Atrio-ventricular (AV) fistula is the anastomosis of an artery and a vein for purposes of haemodialysis in patients with renal failure. It provides access for the artificial kidney machine.

**AV node**   *Quick Reference:* Atrio-ventricular node of the heart.

*Advanced Reference:* Node situated between the atria and ventricles which transmits impulses and forms a pathway in the cardiac conduction system.

**Avulsion**   *Quick Reference:* (avul-shon) To tear away.

*Advanced Reference:* Indicates to forcibly wrench away, as in avulsion of toe-nail when just the nail is removed but not including the bed. Also, avulsion of *varicose veins*.

**Ayre's T-piece**   *Quick Reference:* (airs) Paediatric anaesthetic circuit.

*Advanced Reference:* Corresponds to the *Mapleson* E system. Suitable for children up to 20 kg. The *Jackson Rees* modification added an open-ended bag with an open tail and this enables artificial ventilation.

# B

**Babcock**  *Quick Reference:* A tissue-holding forceps used during bowel surgery.

*Advanced Reference:* A hollow-ended holder that can pick up bowel without damage to the delicate bowel tissue.

**Bacillus**  *Quick Reference:* (bas-il-us) Term used originally to mean a rod-shaped, as opposed to a round, micro-organism.

*Advanced Reference:* The many diseases caused by bacilli include anthrax, diphtheria, gas gangrene, tetanus, tuberculosis and typhoid.

**Back**  *Quick Reference:* Pertaining to the *posterior* surface.

*Advanced Reference:* Refers to the rear surface of the patients' trunk. Is referred to as the *dorsum* of an anatomical surface. The dorsum (back) of the hand as used for intravenous (IV) cannulation.

**Back bar**  *Quick Reference:* Connecting block that seats the anaesthetic *vaporiser*.

*Advanced Reference:* The back bar is situated between the *flowmeters* and the connecting fresh gas flow pipeline within the anaesthetic machine. Commonly the back bar contains the selectatec seating pins for the vaporiser to be positioned in line. More modern back bars allow for multiple vaporisers to be fitted with interlocking mechanisms designed to prevent simultaneous delivery of vapours.

**Back blows**  *Quick Reference:* Choking airway obstruction relieving method.

*Advanced Reference:* A manoeuvre used as first step in relieving foreign body airway obstruction.

**Back support**  *Quick Reference:* A half-moon-shaped support-offering protection for the patient in the lateral position.

*Advanced Reference:* A back support often termed *lumbar* support is used to support the patient on the operating table. A patient in the lateral position can be precarious and requires the patient to be protected from falling off the operating table. A table clamp holds the support in place. The support has an adjustable arm with antistatic padding covering the metal area.

**Bacteria**   *Quick Reference:* A single cell microbe that has the capacity to multiply.

*Advanced Reference:* Bacteria can become harmful to humans through the increase in number of bacterial cells. Bacteria spread requires food substance, warm temperature and, for some types, the presence of oxygen. Common forms of bacteria are cocci, bacilli and spirochaetes. Through these bacterial forms poisonous toxins are spread via exotoxins (which freely diffuse outward from the bacterial cell and spread throughout the human body) and endotoxins (which are released once the bacteria itself has become dysfunctional).

**Bacterial filter**   *Quick Reference:* A filter attached to the patient's end of a breathing circuit preventing spread of infection.

*Advanced Reference:* Bacterial filters are used more routinely to prevent expired bacteria being transmitted into a breathing system that will later be attached to other patients. The filter contains a 22-mm male and female connector allowing connection between the breathing circuit and the patient airway device.

**Bain breathing system**   *Quick Reference:* A breathing system used in conjunction with an anaesthetics machine.

*Advanced Reference:* A breathing system that attaches to the fresh gas outlet (22 mm connection) comprised of a re-breathing bag at the machine's end along with an expiratory valve. The system has two tubings (co-axial); the inner one being thinner than the outer (red, green, blue or black). The inner tubing carries fresh gas flow to the patient and the outer expired gas which is regulated by the expiratory valve. Equates to the Mapleson D classification.

**Bair hugger**   *Quick Reference:* (bare) A warming device used to regulate and maintain patient's body temperature intraoperatively.

*Advanced Reference:* Bair hugger is the manufacturers name for a paper and plastic blanket that fills with regulated hot area. The movement of hot air within this device flows readily through the blanket offering a constant volume of warm air.

**Bakers cyst**   *Quick Reference:* A cyst found in the *popliteal* space.

*Advanced Reference:* Formed of synovial fluid that has escaped from the bursa, usually secondary to some other condition.

**Balfour retractor**   *Quick Reference:* (bal-for) A self-retaining *retractor* used regularly in abdominal surgery.

*Advanced Reference:* Is of open-ended design with curved, fixed retractor blades and a third centre blade. There is an option to use the centred blade. The blade is attached and screwed into position holding the retractor firmly *in situ* at the operation site. The third blade resembles a *Doyens* retractor, with features of a curved shape and a lip on the underside.

**Balken frame**  *Quick Reference:* Also referred to as Balkan beam. A traction device used in orthopaedics.

*Advanced Reference:* A rectangular frame that fixes to the bed and is used for attaching splints, suspending or changing the position of immobilised limbs or providing continuous traction with weights and pulleys.

**Balloon pump**  *Quick Reference:* Device used to support cardiac output.

*Advanced Reference:* The balloon is positioned within the descending aorta at the beginning of diastole and deflated immediately before systole. Introduced via the femoral artery and inflated with helium or carbon dioxide. Synchronised with the electrocardiography (ECG) and arterial trace. Increases coronary tissue blood flow and improves oxygen supply to the myocardium. A temporary measure in left ventricular failure, cardiogenic shock, after *myocardial infarction* (MI) and pre- or post-cardiac surgery.

**Banding**  *Quick Reference:* Rubber-band ligation.

*Advanced Reference:* The application of a small silastic band, commonly used in *haemorrhoidectomy*, placed around the pedicle of each haemorrhoid.

**Bar**  *Quick Reference:* Unit of pressure.
*Advanced Reference:* $100\,kPa = 1\,bar = 1\,atm = 15\,lb/in^2 = 760\,mmHg$.

**Barbiturate**  *Quick Reference:* Group of drugs used mainly as sedatives and anaesthetics.

*Advanced Reference:* Group of drugs derived from barbituric acid, with a wide range of essentially depressant action. Work by direct action on the brain. *Thiopentone* is the most commonly used barbiturate anaesthetic induction agent.

**Bard Parker**  *Quick Reference:* A surgical blade holder.

*Advanced Reference:* Often referred to as the Bard Parker handle. Bard Parker handles come in different lengths and hold different sizes of surgical blades.

**Barium**  *Quick Reference:* (bare-e-um) A flexible soft silvery metallic element.

*Advanced Reference:* The properties of barium allow it to be detected by X-rays. Barium is used within the X-ray departments as a 'barium meal' for the patient to ingest and it provides a diagnosis of any changes in the digestive system using X-ray images. Barium enema is also used for visualisation of the colon and to impregnate devices entering the body (such as IV *cannulae*, etc.) so as to make them X-ray detectable.

**Barre–Guillain syndrome**  *Quick Reference:* A condition that causes paralysis of the nervous system.

*Advanced Reference:* The disorder encourages the body's immune system to attack the peripheral nervous system. This attack causes a varying degree of tingling sensations, usually commencing in the arms and legs then spreading throughout the body. The condition is life threatening and can cause total paralysis leaving the patient hospitalised and on a life-support machine.

**Bartholin's glands**   *Quick Reference:* A pair of glands one on each side of the opening of the vagina that secrete a lubricant.

*Advanced Reference:* Situated in the labia majora, with their ducts opening outside the vulva. These glands can become infected and cause a painful abscess (Bartholin cyst).

**Baseline**   *Quick Reference:* The normal value of a reading.

*Advanced Reference:* Baseline readings can apply to the initial physiological parameters of a patient before surgical, medical or anaesthetic interventions.

**Basilic**   *Quick Reference:* (bas-il-ic) A prominent vein that runs along the back of the forearm.

*Advanced Reference:* A vein on the inner side of the arm at the bend of the elbow and is sometimes chosen for venepuncture.

**Basket**   *Quick Reference:* A Dormia basket is a surgical instrument designed for stone removal.

*Advanced Reference:* Dormia baskets are used during urological procedures with a cystoscope to retrieve ureteric stones.

**Bassini's operation**   *Quick Reference:* Reconstruction of the inguinal canal.

*Advanced Reference:* Carried out during an inguinal hernia repair.

**BAWO:**   *Quick Reference:* Bilateral antrum wash-out.

*Advanced Reference*: Involves inserting a cannula under the inferior turbinate in order to flush out fluid, pus, etc. from the maxillary sinus, using saline.

**BCC**   *Quick Reference:* Basal cell carcinoma.

*Advanced Reference*: May appear as a nodule or as a small, unstable ulcerating area with persistent crusting. Depending on size, it may be removed under local or general anaesthetic (LA and GA, respectively).

**Beer's knife**   *Quick Reference:* A triangular-shaped knife used in eye surgery.

*Advanced Reference:* The Beer's knife has similarities to a diamond knife. Essentially the knife is used to make an incision into the cornea. The curve-shaped incision allows access for removal and replacement of the lens of the eye. It is named after a German ophthalmologist, G.J. Beer, of the 18th century.

**Belfast roller**   *Quick Reference:* A patient transfer device.

*Advanced Reference*: A board-like device that contains rollers of approximately 8 ft long, covered with black rubber that rotated on the rollers.

The device was inserted under the patient and a draw sheet, which was pulled by staff and the roller effect transferred the patient onto the receiving surface. Taken out of use in the 1980s, claims were made that the metal rollers caused damage to bony prominences.

**Belladonna**   *Quick Reference:* Name of a plant and of the alkaloids produced from it.

*Advanced Reference:* **Atropine** and *hyoscine* are the two most well-known drugs from this source.

**Bellows**   *Quick Reference:* A black concertina cylindrical-shaped rubber device, associated with breathing, contained within a mechanical ventilator.

*Advanced Reference:* Bellows are the extendable rubber aspect of mechanical ventilators that indicate delivered gas volume to the patient. Present on most ventilators, e.g. *Manley, East Radcliffe*, etc.

**Bell's palsy**   *Quick Reference:* Paralysis that occurs down the side of the face.

*Advanced Reference:* Bell's palsy occurs due to oedema being present around the facial nerve or during facial surgery or by accidental pressure placed on the patients' face while in the prone position.

**Benign**   *Quick Reference:* (ben-ine) A non-life-threatening tumour that is treatable.

*Advanced Reference:* A tumour or stricture that is present and treatable. Usually localised and has not spread to other aspects of the body. Benign tumours in the oesophagus on X-ray show a distinct tapering shape compared to *malignant* tumours showing a significant shape with no tapering.

**Bennett's fracture**   *Quick Reference:* Fracture of the thumb.

*Advanced Reference:* Associated with accidental injury by falling onto the adducted thumb towards the palm of the hand. Bennett's fracture describes the initial dislocation of the metacarpal from its base location and a triangular section of the base becomes detached. Treatment involves traction of the thumb and direct pressure on the base to realign the bone fragments, followed by application of a *plaster of Paris* cast (or scotch cast). Removal of the cast usually occurs around the 4–6-week period.

**Benzocaine**   *Quick Reference:* (ben-zo-cane) A *topical anaesthetic* or surface applied Local Anaesthetic (LA).

*Advanced Reference:* A derivative of *lignocaine*, LA which can be used on the skin or mucous membrane.

**Benzodiazepines**   *Quick Reference:* (ben-zo-die-az-a-peen) A group of drugs that affects the central nervous system.

*Advanced Reference:* Primarily used as sedatives or hypnotics, e.g. diazepam *nitrazepam* and *lorazepam*.

**Beta-blocker**  *Quick Reference:* (beeta-blocker) Medications whose effect is to reduce the rate and force of the heartbeat.

*Advanced Reference:* Beta-blocker drugs oppose certain actions of the *sympathetic nervous system* in particular stimulation of the heart. Principally used to treat **hypertension**.

**Betadine**  *Quick Reference:* (bet-a-deen) A skin preparation or a surgical scrub solution.

*Advanced Reference:* Betadine is a trade name for an iodine-based solution. Iodine is used to minimise the spread of bacteria on the skin surface. Betadine can be clearly identified by its unique dark yellow/brown appearance.

**Bevan report**  *Quick Reference:* Government commissioned report into the staffing of operating theatres.

*Advanced Reference:* Professor Gilroy Bevan found that there were difficulties within theatre when one group of staff (anaesthesia or surgery) may be absent causing cancellation of operating lists. Skill mix and multi-skilling soon became a focused concern following the report.

**Biceps**  *Quick Reference:* (bi-seps) Main muscle of the upper section of the arm.

*Advanced Reference:* Biceps are connected to the shoulder joint and held to the radius by tendons. They participate in the mechanics of lifting of the forearm by counteracting the action of the triceps.

**Biconcave**  *Quick Reference:* (buy-con-cave) A structure that has inwardly curved depressions on both sides.

*Advanced Reference:* The inwardly facing structures often present themselves in various pieces of equipment as transmitters of light from one focal point to another.

**Biconvex**  *Quick Reference:* A structure that has outward curvatures.

*Advanced Reference:* Can be found as with biconcave structures in devices that transmit light.

**Bicuspid**  *Quick Reference:* Indicates having two projections or cusps.

*Advanced Reference:* The mitral valve of the heart between the left atrium and ventricle is also known as a bicuspid valve due to its significant shape.

**Bier's block**  *Quick Reference:* (beers) Regional analgesia technique used on limbs.

*Advanced Reference:* Bier's block is a Local Anaesthetic (LA) technique used primarily for upper limbs and to a lesser extent legs. Involves use of a double (tourniquet) cuff. The *proximal* cuff is inflated followed by LA injected into a vein, once the local starts to work the distal cuff is inflated and when fully inflated the *proximal* cuff is deflated. The distal cuff would thus be over an area that is affected by the LA.

**Bifid**  *Quick Reference:* The separation of a structure into two parts.

*Advanced Reference:* Often referred to as cleft. Commonly associated with *cleft palate.* Also, a bifid uterus.

**Bifurcate**  *Quick Reference:* (bi-for-cate) The division of a structure into two branches.

*Advanced Reference:* Arteries and veins continually bifurcate throughout the human body. The trachea bifurcates into two main *bronchi.* The bifurcation point of the trachea is known as the *carina.*

**Bigeminy**  *Quick Reference:* (buy-gem-iny) Bi indicates two. Refers to a cardiac dysrhythmia/arrhythmia.

*Advanced Reference:* Term that refers to ectopic beats seen on an ECG trace and when they appear in pairs.

**Bilateral**  *Quick Reference:* (bi-lat-eral) Refers to both sides.

*Advanced Reference:* Bi meaning two, is applied to surgery by stating that both sides of a structure will be operated upon. Bilateral inguinal hernia repair, means the patient has an inguinal hernia of both sides of the abdomen and will be repaired under one anaesthetic.

**Bile**  *Quick Reference:* A liquefied enzyme that is secreted by the liver.

*Advanced Reference:* A yellow-green-coloured sticky fluid that becomes concentrated in the storage pouch of the biliary tree, i.e. the *gall bladder.* The substance travels from the gall bladder along the *cystic duct* down through the *common bile duct* and into the *duodenum.* The main function of bile is to assist in the breakdown of emulsifying fats and may be seen within the *naso-gastric tube* when inserted into patients undergoing gastric surgery.

**Biliary tree**  *Quick Reference:* Refers to the components associated with production and passage of *bile.*

*Advanced Reference:* The main components of the biliary tree are the liver, gall bladder, cystic duct, common bile duct the *ampulla of vater,* head of *pancreas* and associated arteries and veins.

**Bilirubin**  *Quick Reference:* Orange-coloured substance produced by the destruction of *haem.*

*Advanced Reference:* Bilirubin is circulated to the liver within the plasma cells later to be filtered by the liver and eventually excreted in the bile. The accumulation of bilirubin in the blood and tissues results in the yellow pigmentation of the patients' skin and eyes. This discolouration is associated with jaundice.

**Billroth**  *Quick Reference:* A type of *gastrectomy.*

*Advanced Reference:* Named after an Austrian surgeon who developed the technique of removing the majority of the lesser curvature of the stomach and the pyloric segment. The remaining section of the fundus and antrum of the stomach are then *anastomosed* to the *duodenum.*

**Bimetallic strip**   *Quick Reference:* A temperature-compensating device within modern vaporisers.

*Advanced Reference:* A bimetallic strip containing two dissimilar metals that are fused together and expand at different rates when heat is applied. If one metal is heated and starts to expand, the other counter-acts and prevents full expansion of the other. This process is utilised in vaporisers to maintain the regulated percentage of volatile being delivered, irrespective of surrounding temperature changes.

**Bio-hazard**   *Quick Reference:* Any hazard arising from inadvertent human biological processes.

*Advanced Reference:* Examples would be, needle-stick injuries, spillages (chemicals, body fluids, etc.).

**Biopsy**   *Quick Reference:* Small sample of tissue for study.

*Advanced Reference:* Biopsies are usually taken for study under a microscope and can assist with the diagnosis of a patient's condition or underlying disease. There are different types of biopsy, e.g. Trucut biopsy, frozen section. Often referred to as 'taking a bite'.

**Bipolar**   *Quick Reference:* Device or structure with two poles.

*Advanced Reference:* Often referred to, in theatre, as bipolar diathermy. Bipolar diathermy being that the current flows down one pole (on the forceps) and travels back up the second pole. Also used in psychiatry to describe certain conditions.

**Birketts**   *Quick Reference:* Long curved artery forceps.

*Advanced Reference:* Fine curved tip artery forceps that are used during abdominal surgery. The fine tips are useful to clamp vessels and struc-tures, when dissecting the mesentery from the intestinal system.

**Birth canal**   *Quick Reference:* Relating to the passage through the uterine cervix.

*Advanced Reference:* The birth canal is the channel formed by the *cervix*, *vagina* and *vulva* through which the *foetus* is expelled during normal birth.

**Bispectral index**   *Quick Reference:* A sophisticated electroencephalogram (EEG).

*Advanced Reference:* An EEG machine popular in American anaesthe-sia and used to monitor the activities of the brain. By placing the elec-trodes onto the patient's head the anaesthetist can monitor the effects of anaesthesia and interpret these in relation to awareness.

**Bite guard**   *Quick Reference:* Used to protect the patients' teeth.

*Advanced Reference:* Bite guards are made of silicone/rubber and can be used while intubating or during electro-convulsive therapy (*ECT*). The bite guard is essentially intended to prevent damage to teeth, tongue and lips, etc.

**Bladder** *Quick Reference:* A sac or container able to hold a volume of fluid.
*Advanced Reference:* Bladder is often described in theatre in relation to two anatomical structures of the human body: (1) Urinary bladder, Part of the renal system where the ureters from the right and left kidneys drain into. The bladder becomes the collection chamber for urine. (2) The *gall bladder* within the biliary system acting as a collection chamber for bile excreted from the liver.

**Blade** *Quick Reference:* Refers to *scalpel* blade.
*Advanced Reference* Blades come in different sizes and shapes, and are attached to a compatible handle such as a *Bard Parker handle*. Also refers to disposable scalpels.

**Bleeder** *Quick Reference:* A bleeding vessel.
*Advanced Reference:* Slang term that refers to a damaged blood vessel usually during surgery.

**Blepharoplasty** *Quick Reference:* (blef-row-plasty) Correction of excessive tissue of the eyelids.
*Advanced Reference:* Operation performed to reduce the excess tissue from the upper and lower eyelids. Excess tissue occurs often during the ageing process. Termed as a plastic or cosmetic operation.

**Blood** *Quick Reference:* A red fluid contained within the vessels.
*Advanced Reference:* Blood circulates through the heart and blood vessels supplying oxygen and nutrients to all parts of the body. Consists of approximately 55% fluid and 45% cells, etc. Adult volume is about 5 l. Blood plasma is the fluid part of the blood in which the cells are suspended and the fluid left after the blood has clotted is called *serum*. Blood flow is defined as perfusion pressure (over) resistance.

**Blood–brain barrier** *Quick Reference:* The membrane between the blood and the brain.
*Advanced Reference:* A permeable membrane that supports movement of water, oxygen, carbon dioxide and other substances such as alcohol and GA drugs. Essentially the blood–brain barrier maintains a distinctive separation of the blood from direct contact with the brain but supports the passage of essential components. Often jokingly referred to by anaesthetists as the dividing line (at the screen/towel rail) between surgery and anaesthesia.

**Blood clotting** *Quick Reference:* The solidifying of blood.
*Advanced Reference:* Where blood has started to coagulate to form a jelly-like substance. Clotting can occur external to the blood vessel or even within the vessel. Blood clotting is a natural mechanism of the human body when injury occurs.

**Blood-gas analysis** *Quick Reference:* Blood-gas measurement involves the analysis of heparinised fresh arterial blood.

*Advanced Reference:* The parameters measured are arterial blood oxygen and carbon dioxide partial pressures and the pH of the arterial blood. From these other parameters can be ascertained, e.g. bicarbonate, base excess.

**Blood patch**   *Quick Reference:* Done for the relief of post-spinal headache following dural puncture.

*Advanced Reference:* Injection of 10–20 ml of autologous venous blood, immediately after removal from a peripheral vein into the extradural space. It is performed for the relief of post-spinal headache following dural puncture. Diligent attention to asepsis is observed at all times.

**Blood pressure**   *Quick Reference:* Pressure exerted by the blood on the walls of the blood vessels (arteries).

*Advanced Reference:* Blood is driven through the arteries by pressure. It is highest when the heart contracts (systole) and lowest when it relaxes (diastole). In an adult this is approximately 120 mmHg (systolic) and 80 mmHg (diastolic). Blood pressure alters with disease and age.

**Blood products**   *Quick Reference:* Refers to products present in or obtained from donated blood.

*Advanced Reference:* Plasma reduced blood or packed red cells have had a portion of the plasma removed in order to be used for specific functions, these include fresh-frozen plasma (FFP), platelets, factor VIII, etc.

**Blood sugar**   *Quick Reference:* Amount of glucose in the circulating blood.

*Advanced Reference:* Expressed in millimoles per litre. Normal range is 3.5–5.5 mmol/l.

**Blood transfusion**   *Quick Reference:* The transfer of blood or administering of donated blood.

*Advanced Reference:* May be donated from another person of the same blood grouping or oneself (auto). Involves the introduction of stored or removed blood into the circulatory system via a blood-giving set. Transfusion is carried out for a number of both medical and surgical reasons, e.g. blood loss, anaemia, etc.

**Blood warmer**   *Quick Reference:* Device used for warming transfused blood.

*Advanced Reference:* A number of designs are available; e.g. coil through warmed water, electric element, etc. All designed to prevent the adverse effects of transfused blood taken straight from the fridge.

**BMI**   *Quick Reference:* The body mass index (BMI) of an individual can be used to calculate the obesity risk to health.

*Advanced Reference:* $\text{BMI} = \dfrac{\text{weight (kg)}}{\text{height (m}^2)}$.

**Bobbin**   *Quick Reference:* Constituent part of a gas flowmeter/rotameter.
*Advanced Reference:* The bobbin is the measuring indicator within a flowmeter and alters as the needle valve is adjusted to provide more or less gas. The reading of gas flow is taken as the top of the bobbin.

**Bodok seal**   *Quick Reference:* A rubber seal with an outer metal circumference.
*Advanced Reference:* Bodok seals were first developed by British Oxygen Company (BOC). They were designed primarily as a seal and to prevent friction and build-up pressure between two metal surfaces, i.e. the cylinder and the pin index holder (yoke). The Bodok seal is placed onto the seating of the yoke around the gas outlet port and offered up against the pin index-locating hole on the anaesthetic machine.

**Boiling (water)**   *Quick Reference:* Not considered now as a sterilisation process.
*Advanced Reference:* Is only a method of disinfection as it cannot be guaranteed to kill spores (sporicidal).

**Bolus**   *Quick Reference:* A single one-off dose.
*Advanced Reference:* Bolus can be referred to in two different contexts: (1) A bolus of food that is soft after mastication and swallowed. (2) A bolus for injection describes a single amount of medication given as one dose.

**Bone nibblers**   *Quick Reference:* A surgical instrument may be of heavy or fine design depending on need.
*Advanced Reference:* Used during orthopaedic or neurosurgery to remove (nibble) small pieces of bone.

**Bone wax**   *Quick Reference:* A haemostatic material.
*Advanced Reference:* Used mostly in neuro- and spinal surgery on bleeding cancellous bone surfaces.

**Bougie**   *Quick Reference:* (boo-gee) Intubation aid.
*Advanced Reference:* Name given to a gum-elastic malleable catheter used as an aid in difficult intubation. In the event of poor visualisation during intubation, the bougie is fed via the vocal cords into the trachea and the endotracheal (ET) tube introduced over this.

**Bourdon**   *Quick Reference:* (bur-don) A pressure gauge usually fitted to high-pressure cylinders, e.g. oxygen.
*Advanced Reference:* The gauge works on the bourdon tube principle that when pressure is exerted into the curved tube the end begins to straighten, thus manipulating the rack and the pivotal point of the needle to show the reading on the calibrated markers.

**Bowel**   *Quick Reference:* Referring to the intestines.

*Advanced Reference:* The bowel or intestine is commonly referred either to the small or large intestines. Small bowel comprises the duodenum, jejunum, ileum and terminates at the ileo-caecal valve, this is where the large bowel begins and becomes the ascending colon, transverse colon, descending colon, sigmoid, rectum, terminating with the anus.

**Bowel clamp**   *Quick Reference:* A surgical instrument used to occlude the bowel.

*Advanced Reference:* Bowel clamps are either crushing or non-crushing, and are used in pairs during surgery. Some of the most commonly used being Doyens and Pyres.

**Bowie–Dick test**   *Quick Reference:* A test used to measure the efficiency of an autoclave.

*Advanced Reference:* Prior to the daily use of an autoclave for sterilising of surgical equipment, a Bowie–Dick test is performed. The test consists of a small section of surgical paper and an autoclave tape stretched across all corners to make a large X. This is then inserted between a number of surgical drapes and put into the autoclave. A normal autoclave cycle is run and ideally produces a colour change in the autoclave tape which indicates steam penetration but not sterility.

**Bowman's capsule**   *Quick Reference:* Structure within the kidney nephron proximal to the tubules.

*Advanced Reference:* Opening area of the *nephron*, a cup-shaped structure which surrounds the **glomerulus**.

**Boyle's**   *Quick Reference:* Indicates a number of anaesthetic-related adjuncts and named after Henry Boyle, an English anaesthetist.

*Advanced Reference:* The standard anaesthetic machine is named after him and even the modern, much changed machines are still referred to in this way. Also, the Boyles bottle, which is a simple glass jar acting as a *vaporiser* that allowed the passing of a fresh gas flow over a surface area of volatile liquid. The gas passing over the surface of the liquid would aid vaporisation to take place. To increase the amount of vaporisation taking place, it was found that the surface area of gas to pass over would need to increase. The introduction of wicks and movable plunger meant that the degree of control could be applied offering higher concentrations of volatile agents, i.e. ether.

**Boyle–Davis gag**   *Quick Reference:* Mouth gag used in ear, nose and throat (ENT) and oral surgery.

*Advanced Reference:* Used specifically in tonsillectomy and fitted between the teeth to keep the mouth open. Comes with both split and fixed tongue plates.

**Brachial**   *Quick Reference:* (brake-e-al) Pertaining to the arm.

*Advanced Reference:* In the strict sense is the upper arm, with the brachial artery being the main blood vessel.

**Brachial plexus**   *Quick Reference:* A network of nerves at the root of the neck supplying the upper limbs of the body.

*Advanced Reference:* A complex network of nerves that is formed chiefly by the lower four cervical nerves and the first thoracic nerve, lies partly within the *axilla* and supplies nerves to the chest, shoulder and arm. It is one of the areas of injury risk related to poor patient positioning on the operating table.

**Bradycardia**   *Quick Reference:* Patient (adult) with a slow pulse rate below the level of 60 beats per minute (bpm).

*Advanced Reference:* Brady refers to slow; cardia refers to heart. A bradycardia can occur at any time but must not be confused in a patient, who normally at rest, has a slow pulse, i.e. athletes may have heart rates of 50 bpm or lower.

**Brain**   *Quick Reference:* Central thinking process area contained within the skull.

*Advanced Reference:* The brain is a multifunction organ that has two hemispheres with one for logical thinking and the other for abstract thinking. The brain receives and sends messages to all other systems within the human body. Components of the brain are the cerebrum, midbrain, cerebellum, medulla oblongata and pons varolii.

**Brain stem**   *Quick Reference:* The portion of the spinal system between the brain and the spinal cord.

*Advanced Reference:* Consists of the medulla oblongata, pons and midbrain.

**Breathing systems**   *Quick Reference:* A term that describes the apparatus for gas flow to and from the patient.

*Advanced Reference:* These involve anaesthetic circuits of numerous designs, also those related to ventilators as well as the non-rebreathing types, such as Ambu bag, bagvalve mask (BVM), etc. primarily used in resuscitation.

**Breech**   *Quick Reference:* Buttocks first.

*Advanced Reference:* Applies to the lie/position of the foetus in the uterus when it presents buttocks first rather than the normal position of head first.

**Bretylium**   *Quick Reference:* (bret-eel-eum) An *antihypertensive* and ***antiarrhythmic*** drug, e.g. bretylate.

*Advanced Reference:* Used primarily to treat cardiac dysrhythmias and tachycardia.

**Brietal**   *Quick Reference:* Anaesthetic induction agent, e.g. methohexitone.
*Advanced Reference:* Short-acting barbiturate induction agent available as a powder for reconstitution into a 1% solution. Caused hiccoughing and contraindicated in epilepsy. Mostly been replaced by diprivan (propofol).

**Broad ligaments**   *Quick Reference:* Ligaments related to attachment of the female uterus.
*Advanced Reference:* The broad ligaments support the blood vessels to the uterus and uterine tubes and consist of folds of peritoneum which extend from the uterus to the sides of the pelvis.

**Bronchial blocker**   *Quick Reference:* Term also used to indicate endo-bronchial and double-lumen tubes such as Robert-Shaw, Gordon-Green and Carlins tubes.
*Advanced Reference:* Used in thoracic surgery to isolate either lung or portion of.

**Bronchodilator**   *Quick Reference:* (bronco-die-lator) Any agent that relaxes the smooth muscles of the bronchial passages.
*Advanced Reference:* There are many causes of spasm in the bronchial muscles; most common are *asthma* and bronchitis. The best known and most used are *salbutamol* and *aminophylline*.

**Bronchopleural fistula**   *Quick Reference:* (bronco-plural) Abnormal connection between the tracheobronchial tree and the pleura.
*Advanced Reference:* Occurs after surgery (*pneumonectomy*), following trauma, infection or damage due to a tumour.

**Bronchoscopy**   *Quick Reference:* Procedure for visually examining the trachea and main bronchus and lung.
*Advanced Reference:* Carried out using either fibre-optic or rigid bronchoscope. Usually carried out under GA when ventilation is maintained using a *Venturi* injector.

**Bronchospasm**   *Quick Reference:* (bron-co-spasm) Narrowing of the bronchi.
*Advanced Reference:* Narrowing is due to muscular contraction due to a stimulus as in *asthma* and bronchitis. Relieved with *bronchodilator* drugs.

**Bronchus**   *Quick Reference:* (bron-cus) Windpipe or bronchial tube.
*Advanced Reference:* The bronchi refers to either of the two primary divisions of the trachea that lead, respectively, into the right and left lung.

**Brooks airway**   *Quick Reference:* Type of oropharyngeal airway.
*Advanced Reference:* An airway designed for use in mouth-to-mouth resuscitation but allows for non-contact between rescuer and victim. It has a mouth guard/cover which is designed to form an airtight seal.

**Brown fat** *Quick Reference:* Specialised adipose tissue involved in the generation of heat.

*Advanced Reference:* Of special importance in neonates. Distributed throughout the body (mainly in upper back and shoulder area) of the newborn, it allows for increase in the metabolism and thus heat production, while simultaneously using up the fat itself.

**Buccal** *Quick Reference:* (book-al) Pertaining to the mouth or cheek.

*Advanced Reference:* The buccal cavity is the mouth and consists of two parts: the outer or vestibule, which is the space outside of the teeth and within the lips and cheeks, and the inner part which communicates with the oropharynx.

**Buffer** *Quick Reference:* A solution in which the concentration of hydrogen ions remains constant despite the addition of an **alkali** or acid.

*Advanced Reference:* **Sodium bicarbonate** is the body's chief buffering system.

**Bulldog** *Quick Reference:* A vascular clamp.

*Advanced Reference:* A small vascular clamp designed to hold the vessel securely but without causing trauma. All bulldog clamps must be counted and recorded within the instrument count.

**Bundle branch block** *Quick Reference:* An irregularity in the cardiac conduction system.

*Advanced Reference:* Involves a delay in conduction along either side (left or right) of the atrio-ventricular (AV) bundle and related to **heart block**. Detected on an ECG trace.

**Bundle of His** *Quick Reference:* Large collection of *neuromuscular* fibres that pass through the middle of the heart (**septum**).

*Advanced Reference:* The beginning of the bundle of His starts with the AV node that collects the electrical activity caused by the **sino-atrial node**. The electrical current is transmitted down and through the fibres and then brings about contraction within the ventricles.

**Bung** *Quick Reference:* A rubber end or plastic cap that is used to close off the end of an IV line.

*Advanced Reference:* Bung can be found in the end of blood specimen bottles. *Leur lock* caps can be referred to as a bung.

**Bunion** *Quick Reference:* A deformity of the joint at the base of the big toe.

*Advanced Reference:* Caused by friction and pressure from shoes, forming a bursa. Severe forms require surgery, with the operation being termed hallux valgus. A bursa is a fibrous sac lined with synovial membrane and contains a small quantity of synovial fluid.

B

**Bupivacaine**   *Quick Reference:* (bu-piv-a-cane) A Local Anaesthetic (LA) agent that has a longer action than *lignocaine*.

*Advanced Reference:* Bupivacaine has a slow onset of action but has the distinct advantage of lasting longer than most alternative LAs. Often used for skin infiltration around the wound site to give a degree of pain relief for the patient following surgery. *Heavy marcain* a form of bupivaine with *glucose* is used during spinal anaesthesia.

**Burette**   *Quick Reference:* (be-yur-et) Piece of IV infusion equipment.

*Advanced Reference:* Involves a measuring chamber which attaches into the IV bag or giving set allowing monitoring of infusion volume. Used when volume and dose are critical, e.g. paediatric infusion and/or drug administration.

**Burr**   *Quick Reference:* Surgical drill bit.

*Advanced Reference:* Used for drilling or cutting bone or teeth.

**Burr hole**   *Quick Reference:* Holes drilled in the cranium.

*Advanced Reference:* Carried out to gain access to the brain or release pressure inside the *cranium.*

**Bursa**   *Quick Reference:* Small fibrous sac containing synovial fluid.

*Advanced Reference:* Intended to reduce friction where structures move over one another, i.e. around joints, between a tendon and a bone, although they can also be formed in some locations by friction and pressure.

**Buscopan**   *Quick Reference:* Antispasmodic drug used to relax the intestinal wall.

*Advanced Reference:* Buscopan is the trade name of *hyoscine* butylbromide. The drug is usually given 20–30 min prior to a patient having a gastroscopy or a sigmoidoscopy. Relaxing the intestines allows greater flexibility for the scope to be advanced through the intestinal system avoiding trauma. Provides for a lighter relief of pain during the diagnostic investigation.

**Butterfly needle**   *Quick Reference:* A type of IV needle.

*Advanced Reference:* Has plastic sides which act as a grip for insertion and lie flat on the skin for fixation once sited. Available in a range of gauges.

**BVM**   *Quick Reference:* Abbreviation for bagvalve mask, which is a self-inflating breathing circuit.

*Advanced Reference:* Used mainly for resuscitation purposes, has more or less replaced the *Ambu bag.*

**Bypass**   *Quick Reference:* Indicates diversion of flow as from the normal route.

*Advanced Reference:* Can refer to cardiopulmonary bypass as used in cardiac surgery, aorta bi-femoral bypass in vascular surgery, and use of a shunt in carotid artery bypass.

**CABG**   *Quick Reference:* Coronary artery bypass graft. Referred to as 'cabbage'.
   *Advanced Reference:* A surgical procedure to bypass diseased or damaged coronary arteries using the patient's own veins, usually the saphenous of the leg.

**Cadaver**   *Quick Reference:* A corpse.
   *Advanced Reference:* Refers to a dead body used for dissection or harvesting of organs.

**Caecum**   *Quick Reference:* (see-come) First part of the large intestine.
   *Advanced Reference:* It lies in the lower right side of the abdominal cavity. The appendix opens off the caecum.

**Caesarean section**   *Quick Reference:* Delivery of a baby through an abdominal incision.
   *Advanced Reference:* Performed for a variety of reasons and conditions, e.g. foetal distress, placenta previa, etc. There still remains debate about the origins of the title. One view is that Julius Caesar was born via this method, another states that it stems from a law or dictate issued by Caesar proclaiming that all women dying during childbirth should be cut open in order to save the life of the baby.

**Calcium**   *Quick Reference:* Metallic element.
   *Advanced Reference:* Calcium levels in the blood are approximately 0.01%. Deficiency or excess can seriously disturb the function of nerve cells and muscle fibres also being necessary in the blood-clotting process. Correct concentration is maintained by the action of hormones of the *parathyroid glands*.

**Calcium antagonist**   *Quick Reference:* Group of drugs used as antihypertensives.
   *Advanced Reference:* Used in the treatment of hypertension. They act by reducing calcium entry into the heart which reduces the force of the heartbeat and therefore lowers blood pressure (BP).

C

**Calculi**   *Quick Reference:* Commonly referred to as stones.

*Advanced Reference:* An abnormal and excessive accumulation of mineral salts.

**Calculus**   *Quick Reference:* (Calculi) A hard insoluble mass (stone) in any hollow organ.

*Advanced Reference:* Calculi are formed from substances normally dissolved in the fluid contents of the organ, e.g. kidneys, urinary bladder, gall bladder, salivary glands.

**Caldwell-Luc**   *Quick Reference:* Surgical operation to drain the maxillary sinus.

*Advanced Reference:* Also referred to as antrostomy. An artificial opening is made through the upper jaw opposite the second molar tooth.

**Calibrate**   *Quick Reference:* To calculate, correlate readings with a standard.

*Advanced Reference:* Can refer to calibration of manometers, etc. A transducer used for invasive central venous pressure (*CVP*)/arterial readings, calibrated to atmosphere before connecting to a patient so to set a constant standard for readings.

**Caliper**   *Quick Reference:* Two pronged device used to exert traction.

*Advanced Reference:* Used as part of traction apparatus with fractures, especially those of the power limb. Also a measuring device/instrument.

**Callus**   *Quick Reference:* Hard tissue formed at the site of a broken bone.

*Advanced Reference:* Callus collects around and between the bone ends. Cells called osteoblasts multiply and form irregular bone which knits the ends together as new bone develops.

**Calorie**   *Quick Reference:* Unit of energy.

*Advanced Reference:* Is the amount of heat required to warm 1 kg of water by 1°C. The calorie value of food is the number of calories it would yield if it were completely burnt.

**Canal**   *Quick Reference:* Passageway.

*Advanced Reference:* Examples are the anal canal, alimentary canal.

**Cancer**   *Quick Reference:* A disorder of cell growth.

*Advanced Reference:* A carcinogen is any substance liable to cause cancer. The term carcinoma is used generally but actually indicates cancers arising in or covering membranes.

**Candela**   *Quick Reference:* SI unit of luminosity.

*Advanced Reference:* A measure of the intensity of luminosity.

**Cannulation**   *Quick Reference:* To make access to a vessel, etc. with a cannula.

*Advanced Reference:* Term most commonly used in relation to the insertion of intravenous (IV) cannulae. Can however also indicate access to an artery and several other invasive techniques. Often used interchangeably with catheterisation, but this commonly indicates a longer device, i.e. *CVP* or as in bladder catheterisation of the *urethra*.

**Capacitance** *Quick Reference:* To store; stored electrical charge.

*Advanced Reference:* Something with the ability to retain an electrical charge. A capacitor consists of a conductor separated by an insulator and so prevents (stores) flow of direct current (DC) and maintains it ready for discharge. A defibrillator is charged to the required joules ready to deliver the shock and the capacitor stores the energy which is then delivered as/when required.

**Capillary** *Quick Reference:* Smallest blood vessel.

*Advanced Reference:* A minute vessel which connects an arteriole and a venule. It is in the capillary that the blood and the tissue fluids exchange gases, food and waste products.

**Capnograph** *Quick Reference:* A device which displays *carbon dioxide* ($CO_2$) concentration.

*Advanced Reference:* Capnography utilises infrared light absorption to measure $CO_2$ concentration, most commonly end-tidal $CO_2$ when it is displayed in both numerical and wave form. End-tidal $CO_2$ approximates to alveolar $PCO_2$ which in turn indicates arterial $PCO_2$. Capnometry indicates measurement only or the reading of $CO_2$.

**Capsule** *Quick Reference:* Fibrous *sheath* enclosing an organ.

*Advanced Reference:* The tough flexible casing of a joint strengthened with ligaments and lined with a synovial membrane.

**Carbolic acid** *Quick Reference:* Phenol.

*Advanced Reference:* One of the first antiseptics. Still used as a standard to measure newer *germicides*.

**Carbon** *Quick Reference:* Non-metallic chemical element.

*Advanced Reference:* At one time operating table covers, wheels, anaesthetic tubing, etc. contained carbon as a conductor for static electricity.

**Carbon dioxide** *Quick Reference:* Colourless gas which comprises 0.03% of air. Product of body metabolism. Chemical symbol $CO_2$.

*Advanced Reference:* Formed following oxygen metabolism in the body and carried via the blood and plasma in the veins to the lungs where it forms approximately 3–4% of expired air. When dissolved in water, forms carbonic acid and it is carried mainly in this state to the lungs.

**Carbon monoxide** *Quick Reference:* Colourless, odourless gas formed by the incomplete burning of fuels. Most common example is car-exhaust fumes.

*Advanced Reference:* It combines with the haemoglobin much easier than oxygen and leads to carbon monoxide poisoning which is a type of asphyxia. However, it produces a bright pink complexion rather than the blue appearance associated with the lack of oxygen.

**Carcinoma**  *Quick Reference:* From the Greek Karkinoma and karkinos (crab). Used as a term to denote *cancer*.
  *Advanced Reference:* A malignant growth made up of epithelial cells tending to infiltrate the surrounding tissues.

**Cardex**  *Quick Reference:* Surgeon and anaesthetist preference cards.
  *Advanced Reference:* System for recording both surgeon and anaesthetist requirements for individual procedures.

**Cardiac arrest**  *Quick Reference:* Cessation of the heartbeat.
  *Advanced Reference:* Indicates sudden circulatory stoppage. Signs and symptoms include absent pulse, apnoea, cyanosis. Treatment is immediate institution of cardiopulmonary resuscitation (*CPR*).

**Cardiac catheterisation**  *Quick Reference:* Passage of a catheter under radiographical control through an artery or vein until it reaches the heart.
  *Advanced Reference:* Used in the diagnosis and study of heart disease and related conditions.

**Cardiac cycle**  *Quick Reference:* A sequence of events lasting about 0.8 s.
  *Advanced Reference:* The cardiac cycle occurs when the atria and ventricles contract thus forcing blood around the body. Each cycle lasting about 0.8 s.

**Cardiac massage**  *Quick Reference:* Manual compression of the heart.
  *Advanced Reference:* Rhythmic compression of the heart performed in order to re-establish circulation usually after cardiac arrest. Can be performed externally or internally.

**Cardiac output**  *Quick Reference:* Volume of blood expelled from the heart each minute.
  *Advanced Reference:* Is dependent on stroke volume and heart rate. Cardiac output = stroke volume (l) × heart rate (bpm), where bpm is beats per minute.

**Cardiology**  *Quick Reference:* Branch of physiology and medicine concerned with the heart.
  *Advanced Reference:* A cardiologist is a physician who specialises in disease and damage to the heart and surrounding tissue.

**Cardiomyopathy**  *Quick reference:* A chronic disorder of the heart muscle.
  *Advanced Reference:* A general diagnostic term designating a primary disease of the heart muscle often of obscure or unknown origin.

**Cardiopulmonary**  *Quick Reference:* Relating to the heart and lungs.
  *Advanced Reference:* Term applied to many activities and situations, e.g. *CPR*, cardiopulmonary bypass refers to use of a heart–lung machine during open heart surgery.

**Cardiovascular**  *Quick Reference:* Terminology relating to the heart and blood vessels.

*Advanced Reference:* Referring to the pulmonary and systemic circulation and the network of arteries and veins throughout the body.

**Cardioversion**  *Quick Reference:* Application of synchronised DC electric current to restore *sinus rhythm.*

*Advanced Reference:* Use of the *defibrillator* at varying energy levels to treat atrial flutter / fibrillation, ventricular tachycardia and supraventricular *tachycardia* (SVT). The machine is synchronised to deliver the shock to occur with the R-wave of the electrocardiogram (ECG). Delivering the shock during the repolarisation phase can lead to ventricular fibrillation (VF).

**Care pathway**  *Quick Reference:* A hospital-wide multi-disciplinary approach to patient care. Standardised care.

*Advanced Reference:* Should involve all disciplines having their specialised part to play in the care pathway during the patient's hospital stay. The mapping of a disease or through the peri-operative period in order to give standardisation for patient care.

**Care plan**  *Quick Reference:* A tool for planning patient care during the peri-operative phase.

*Advanced Reference:* A care plan will help staff assess, plan, implement and evaluate the operative needs of the patient. Each plan giving individual care to all patients.

**Carotid**  *Quick Reference:* Usually refers to the main artery of the head.

*Advanced Reference:* The carotid artery supplies the head and brain with blood. It has two branches, i.e. the external and internal carotid arteries.

**Carpal tunnel**  *Quick Reference:* Syndrome related to the wrist.

*Advanced Reference:* Compression of the median nerve which causes tingling and numbness in the fingers.

**Carter-Braine**  *Quick Reference:* Arm support used during surgery.

*Advanced Reference:* Type of support used for the upper arm when patient is placed in lateral position, e.g. hip replacement, kidney surgery, etc. Precautions should be taken to minimise the risk of the patient touching the metal section of the support.

**Cartilage**  *Quick Reference:* Gristle, a tough supporting tissue.

*Advanced Reference:* The majority of bones are originally formed from cartilage. When the bone is fully developed, the cartilage remains at the bone ends only, where it forms an articulating surface. Often heard as a sport person knee injury.

**Cast**  *Quick Reference:* Piece of material moulded into a required shape.

*Advanced Reference:* Usually refers to a plaster cast or plaster of Paris (POP).

**CAT or CT**  *Quick Reference:* Computerised axial tomography, a CAT scan.

*Advanced Reference:* An image taken to show structures lying in a selected plane in the body.

**Catabolism**   *Quick Reference:* A chemical breakdown of substances in the body.

*Advanced Reference:* A chemical process by which complex substances are broken down to form simpler substances with the release of energy.

**Catalyst**   *Quick Reference:* (cat-a-list) Substance which brings about a chemical change.

*Advanced Reference:* A catalyst brings about a change without itself actually undergoing any change. *Enzymes* are examples of a catalyst.

**Cataract**   *Quick Reference:* Opacity of the lens of the eye.

*Advanced Reference:* Causes dimness of vision and if not treated may lead to complete loss of vision. Involves removal of the lens and with it the ability to focus. Often an artificial lens is implanted in place of the natural one.

**Catgut**   *Quick Reference:* A suture material made from the intestines of a sheep (no longer used since the outbreak of bovine spongiform enchephalopathy (*BSE*)).

*Advanced Reference:* Suture or ligature material, woven into different strengths. It can be plain or treated with chromic acid to make chromic catgut which acts to extend its absorption.

**Catheter**   *Quick Reference:* A tube designed for introduction into a body cavity, etc.

*Advanced Reference:* Often used interchangeably with cannula but while these tend to be shorter devices, catheters tend to be longer, an example is a bladder catheter. They can be made from plastic, rubber, silicone, etc.

**Catheter mount**   *Quick Reference:* Anaesthetic adjunct.

*Advanced Reference:* Connecting tube which is inserted between the endotracheal (ET) tube and patients' breathing circuit.

**Cation**   *Quick Reference:* Ion with a positive charge.

*Advanced Reference:* Due to the positive charge, a cation moves towards a cathode in the presence of an electric field.

**Caudia equina**   *Quick Reference:* Terminal end of the spinal cord.

*Advanced Reference:* Tail-like appendage which contains the bundle of sacral and lumbar nerves.

**Cautery**   *Quick Reference:* An instrument used to seal a bleeding point during surgery.

*Advanced Reference:* A surgical instrument which applies heat to tissues to stop bleeding. May come in various forms, e.g. needle point, loop, knife or ball diathermy. Known as 'Buzz' or 'diathermy forceps'.

**Cavity**   *Quick Reference:* A walled area within the body.
*Advanced Reference:* A confined well-defined space within the body, e.g. the chest cavity, abdominal cavity and pelvic cavity.

**c.c.**   *Quick Reference:* Cubic centimetre.
*Advanced Reference:* As a measurement, millilitre (ml) is the more exact term.

**CCF**   *Quick Reference:* Congestive cardiac failure.
*Advanced Reference:* Describes the state in which there is both right and left ventricular failure with a combination of systemic and pulmonary symptoms.

**CDH**   *Quick Reference:* Congenital dislocation of the hip.
*Advanced Reference:* Deformity resulting from developmental abnormality. Involves failure in development and thus fit/seating of the head of the femur and acetabulum.

**Cefotaxime**   *Quick Reference:* Broad-spectrum antibiotic. Proprietary preparation is called claforan.
*Advanced Reference:* One of the cephalosporins used to treat a wide range of bacterial infections. Cefuroxime is also a cephalosporin and has similar actions and is used in the treatment of upper respiratory tract and urinary tract infections.

**Cell**   *Quick Reference:* A single-cell unit from which the body is made.
*Advanced Reference:* A microscopic single-celled mass made up of protoplasm, a nucleus and cytoplasm, and is able to reproduce itself by *mitosis*.

**Cellulitis**   *Quick Reference:* Inflammation of cellular tissue.
*Advanced Reference:* Commonly due to infection by ***streptococci*** from contaminated wounds. Treated with ***antibiotics*** and/or ***sulphonamides***.

**Celsius**   *Quick Reference:* Scale for measuring temperature.
*Advanced Reference:* Scale originally based on the melting point of ice which was 0° and the boiling point of water, taken to be 100°. Now in universal use and referred to as celsius or centigrade scale.

**Cement**   *Quick Reference:* Refers to bone cement used in orthopaedic surgery.
*Advanced Reference:* Bone cement is not an adhesive but functions by filling up a space and so forming a better mechanical fit. Most common cements are acrylic. Prepared during the operation by mixing a liquid which contains the monomer and a stabiliser with a powder that includes a ***catalyst*** to initiate polymerisation. Also usually included are a ***radio-opaque*** material and an ***antibiotic***. Quite commonly can cause a reaction which may lead to severe *hypotension* upon application.

C

**Cerebellum**   *Quick Reference:* The hindbrain.
*Advanced Reference:* Situated behind the brain stem and is concerned with balance, muscle tone and co-ordination of movement.

**Cerebrovascular accident**   *Quick Reference:* Referred to as a *stroke* or CVA.
*Advanced Reference:* Caused by a haemorrhage, thrombus or embolus where the patient may become paralysed on one side.

**Cerebrum**   *Quick Reference:* The largest part of the brain.
*Advanced Reference:* Includes the two linked cerebral hemispheres but sometimes used to indicate the brain as a whole.

**Cervical**   *Quick Reference:* Of the neck.
*Advanced Reference:* Pertaining to the neck region, e.g. cervical vertebrae/spine.

**Cervical smear**   *Quick Reference:* A special test for women to diagnose cervical carcinoma.
*Advanced Reference:* The removal of cells from the neck of the womb which are then stained and examined under a microscope. This test is important for the diagnosis of malignant and pre-malignant cells before symptoms develop.

**Cetrimide**   *Quick Reference:* A detergent with antiseptic properties.
*Advanced Reference:* Cetrimide is often combined with the antiseptic *chlorhexidine* and used as a skin preparation.

**Chemotherapy**   *Quick Reference:* A chemical agent used to arrest the progress of or eradicate a disease.
*Advanced Reference:* This group of agents can be administered orally, intramuscularly or intravenous (IV). They are intended to have a desired effect on the diseased area without causing irreversible injury to healthy tissue. Involves mainly the *sulphonamide* and *cytotoxic* groups.

**Cheyne–Stokes respiration**   *Quick Reference:* A pattern of breathing found in patients in a deep coma or dying.
*Advanced Reference:* Instead of a normal breathing rhythm, breaths become deeper/shallower until the breathing stops, then the cycle is repeated.

**Chin support**   *Quick Reference:* Device used to support the chin during general anaesthesia (GA).
*Advanced Reference:* Involves a spatula or similar implement used in conjunction with a harness to support the jaw and maintain the airway during spontaneous breathing mask anaesthesia. Mostly obsolete now due to the use of the laryngeal mask airway (LMA).

**Chlamydia**   *Quick Reference:* (clam-id-ea) Type of micro-organism.
*Advanced Reference:* Classified as a bacteria but has virus-like behaviour in that it can only multiply within cells. Responsible for a number of

diseases, e.g. trachoma, urethritis in men but predominantly associated with cervicitis and salpingitis in women which can lead to infertility. The organism is sensitive to tetracyclines and erythromycin.

**Chloral hydrate** *Quick Reference:* (cloral) Sedative and hypnotic.
*Advanced Reference:* Used orally to induce sleep, mainly with children and the elderly. Can also be administered rectally.

**Chloramphenicol** *Quick Reference:* (clor-am-fen-icol) A broad-spectrum antibiotic, popular in ophthalmics.
*Advanced Reference:* It is administrated topically in the form of eye drops, ear drops, cream or in tablet form.

**Chlorhexidine** *Quick Reference:* An antimicrobial solution used to prevent bacteria multiplying.
*Advanced Reference:* Chlorhexidine forms the basis of handwashing solution and skin preparation fluid within the theatre. It is often seen in a pink colour form that can be applied to the skin. Once applied, if an alcohol based solution, the skin should be allowed to dry preventing any pooling of the solution, which could cause a diathermy risk to the patient.

**Chlorine** *Quick Reference:* An amine found in the body and present in egg yolk and fat. Also a vitamin of the B complex.
*Advanced Reference:* Plays an important part in the metabolism of fats and the functioning of the nervous system in the form of *acetylcholine*.

**Chloroform** *Quick Reference:* A colourless volatile liquid once used for GA.
*Advanced Reference:* Administered as an anaesthetic inhalation agent but no longer in use as it was known to cause heart problems, liver damage and pollution.

**Cholangiogram** *Quick Reference:* X-ray of the biliary tract.
*Advanced Reference:* The introduction of a radio-opaque dye to define the biliary tree and surrounding structures.

**Cholecystectomy** *Quick Reference:* Surgical removal of the gall bladder.
*Advanced Reference:* Usually performed for the removal of symptomatic gall stones and performed most commonly through a right subcostal (*Kochers*) incision or increasingly via a laparoscopic technique.

**Cholecystitis** *Quick Reference:* (colly-sist-itis) Inflammation of the gall bladder.
*Advanced Reference:* Acute pain radiating through to the back causing nausea and vomiting usually due to a stone formation or stones lodged in the cystic duct.

**Cholestasis** *Quick reference:* Stagnation of bile in the *liver*.
*Advanced Reference:* Usually due to obstruction of the bile passages and is a common cause of *jaundice*.

**Cholesterol** *Quick Reference:* Fat-like substance found in most tissues.

*Advanced Reference:* Blood contains about 0.2% cholesterol. Cholesterol is the main component of deposits in the lining of arteries and so associated with *arteriosclerosis.*

**Cholinesterase**   *Quick Reference:* (cole-in-est-erase) Enzyme involved in the formation and destruction of acetylcholine.

*Advanced Reference:* Cholinesterase hydrolyses *acetylcholine* at the neuromuscular junction. Has the same action on *suxamethonium.*

**Chronic**   *Quick Reference:* A disease or condition of long duration.

*Advanced Reference:* Chronic conditions often have a gradual onset. Opposite of acute, which often has a rapid onset but of short duration. Examples would be chronic renal failure and acute renal failure.

**Chyle**   *Quick Reference:* A milky fluid found in the lymphatic system.

*Advanced Reference:* The end product of digested fats which are absorbed through the lymph vessels in the intestinal wall.

**Chyme**   *Quick Reference:* Partly digested stomach contents.

*Advanced Reference:* A semi-liquid acid mass of undigested food that passes into the small intestine.

**Cilia**   *Quick Reference:* Fine hair-like structures.

*Advanced Reference:* Present on the surfaces of certain cells and with an undulating action sweeps matter along body passages, e.g. those of the air passages.

**Circulation**   *Quick Reference:* The flow of blood through the arteries and veins around the body.

*Advanced Reference:* Indicates movement in a circular manner or circuit. Referred to generally as the systemic circulation but should include more accurately the pulmonary, portal, coronary and collateral circulations, each having a specific role. The *pulmonary* involves the passage of blood from the right ventricle through the pulmonary artery, lungs and back to the heart via the pulmonary veins. The *portal* circulation is the passage of the blood from the alimentary tract, pancreas and spleen via the *portal* vein through the *liver* and into the *hepatic* veins. The coronary circulation is the system of vessels which supply the heart muscle itself while the *collateral* indicates the vessels which have the action of establishing a blood flow to an area when the main system fails.

**Circulator**   *Quick Reference:* Refers to the member of staff who provides for the scrub team during surgery. In USA termed scout.

*Advanced Reference:* Indicates someone who moves around and within an activity as opposed to the role of the scrub assistant who by nature is restricted to within the aseptic boundary.

**Circumcision**   *Quick Reference:* Removal of the foreskin of the penis.

*Advanced Reference:* Removal of a part of the foreskin (prepuce) is a better description. Carried out for both medical and religious/cultural reasons. Medical reasons involve *phimosis* and *paraphimosis.*

**Cirrhosis**   *Quick Reference:* (sir-o-sis) Disorder of the liver.
*Advanced reference:* Leads to the development of fibrous tissue in the organ with consequent scarring, hardening and loss of function. There are a number of causes, e.g. chronic alcoholism, chronic *hepatitis* (types B and C).

**Citanest**   *Quick Reference:* Proprietary local anaesthetic (LA).
*Advanced Reference:* It is a preparation of prilocaine hydrochloride. Used regularly as an LA in dental practice. Also available with octapressin as a vasoconstrictor.

**CJD**   *Quick Reference:* Creutzfelds–Jakob disease. A new variant form of 'mad cow' disease also known as *bovine spongiform encephalopathy (BSE).*
*Advanced Reference:* CJD destroys brain cells, leading to confusion, disability and eventually death. It cannot be destroyed by normal sterilisation of surgical instruments. Any instruments used on known infected patients must be removed from use and dealt with according to national policy.

**Clamps**   *Quick Reference:* Generally referring to vascular clamps.
*Advanced Reference:* Specialised instruments used in vascular surgery. They occlude the vessels without causing trauma to the arteries or veins. They are available in many shapes and sizes depending on where in the body they are required. The most popular being Bulldog, Cooley, Debakey, Glover, Leland-Jones and Satinsky, etc.

**Claudication:**   *Quick Reference:* Limping. Name derived from Emperor Claudius who was a cripple.
*Advanced Reference:* Cramp-like pain in the legs during mild exercise due to inadequate blood supply to the muscles from diseased arteries.

**Clausen Head Harness**   *Quick Reference:* A harness used to hold the anaesthetic mask on the patient.
*Advanced Reference:* A three tailed black antistatic harness that assisted the anaesthetist in securing the face mask in position. Although the harness is still available, the laryngeal mask airway has become more popular.

**Clavicle**   *Quick Reference:* The collarbone.
*Advanced Reference:* Bone joined at its inner end to the breastbone and its outer end to the shoulder blade.

**Cleft palate**   *Quick Reference:* Defect in the roof of the mouth.
*Advanced Reference:* Cleft indicates a fissure or opening. A *congenital* condition due to failure of the medial plates of the palate to meet. Has an effect on speech. Often found in conjunction with *harelip.*

**Clinical**   *Quick Reference:* Associated with a clinic, or indicates to the bedside.

C

*Advanced Reference:* Referring to actual observation and treatment of patients, as distinguished from theoretical treatment.

**Clinical trials** *Quick Reference:* Trials carried out in the clinical setting and can involve drugs, equipment, procedures, etc.

*Advanced Reference:* Carried out to determine if a treatment is viable and to make comparisons with current practices.

**Closed circuit** *Quick Reference:* Alternative name used for the circle anaesthetic breathing system.

*Advanced Reference:* So called due to patient re-breathing their own gases as they are recycled via the 'closed' system. Consequently, there is a build-up of carbon dioxide, hence the use of *soda lime* within the circuit as an absorber. Has a number of advantages, i.e. use of low flows therefore reducing pollution and cost, maintains humidification and heat from patients' own expired gases.

**Clostridium** *Quick Reference:* A genus of bacteria.

*Advanced Reference:* Includes those bacteria responsible for tetanus and gas *gangrene*. Are *anaerobic*, i.e. thrive in the absence of oxygen. Most strains of Clostridium are found in soils and infection through this route is common.

**Clubbing** *Quick Reference:* Indicates clubbing of the fingers due to poor circulation.

*Advanced Reference:* Involves both toes and fingers, and due to chronic disease of the heart and respiratory system.

**CNS** *Quick Reference:* Central nervous system.

*Advanced Reference:* Incorporates the spinal cord and brain, and not the peripheral nervous system.

**Coagulation** *Quick Reference:* Refers to the clotting of blood.

*Advanced Reference:* Circulating fibrinogen is converted into insoluble fibrin which forms the framework for a clot. The change from fibrinogen to fibrin is brought about by an enzyme, thrombin, not normally present in normal blood but is produced from prothrombin by the action of thromboplastin which is produced when tissue cells are injured. Platelets (thrombocytes) and calcium are also involved in the clotting process.

**Coarctation** *Quick Reference:* Abnormal narrowing of a vessel.

*Advanced Reference:* The aorta is a common site for this. Often a *congenital* cause and involves constriction which reduces blood flow and supply to those parts downstream of the stricture. Compensation for the blockage involves the establishment of a *collateral* circulation. Surgical intervention is usually required to restore adequate circulation.

**Coaxial** *Quick Reference:* Refers to patient breathing circuits used in anaesthesia where there is more than one channel for inspiration and expiration of gases.

*Advanced Reference:* The most commonly used variations are the Lack and Bain circuits which have two channels. With the former, fresh gas passes via the outer channel carries the fresh gas, and expired gases exit through the inner tube whereas the Bain has the directly opposite arrangement. Corresponds to the Mapleson D arrangement.

**Cocaine**    *Quick Reference: CNS* stimulant.

*Advanced Reference:* Used mainly as an anaesthetic for topical application in ear, nose and throat (ENT) surgery and in eye drops. Once used as a constituent in elixirs prescribed to treat pain in terminal care.

**Coccus**    *Quick Reference:* Spherical-shaped bacteria.

*Advanced Reference:* Cocci are arranged in various groups, i.e. the *Staphylococcus* in bunches like grapes, the *Streptococcus* in chains and the *Diplococcus* in pairs.

**Coccyx**    *Quick Reference:* The lower end of the backbone.

*Advanced Reference:* A small triangular bone projecting beyond the sacrum and consists of four tiny vertebrae fused together. Is all that remains of a human tail.

**Cochlea**    *Quick Reference:* Part of the inner ear.

*Advanced Reference:* Shaped like a spiral shell, the cochlea contains the hearing apparatus. A cochlea implant is an electronic device inserted under GA whose function is to stimulate the auditory nerve in an attempt to restore partial hearing in profound sensory deafness.

**Cockpit drill**    *Quick Reference:* Alternative term used to describe anaesthetic machine checking.

*Advanced Reference:* As the induction and reversal of GA is often likened to the take-off and landing of an aeroplane, the term for checking and preparing anaesthetic equipment was adopted due to the cockpit checks carried out by pilots.

**Codeine**    *Quick Reference:* Alkaloid drug derived from *opium.*

*Advanced Reference:* Closely related to morphine but less powerful and less habit forming. Used for pain relief alone and in combination with other drugs, such as aspirin.

**Coeliac disease**    *Quick Reference:* (seal-e-ac) Disorder of the small intestine.

*Advanced Reference:* Involves malabsorption due to the lining of the intestine not tolerating a component of *gluten* which is a protein found in wheat, barley and rye.

**Colic**    *Quick Reference:* Intermittent pain, often severe, arising from internal organs.

*Advanced Reference:* Due to contraction of involuntary muscles which in turn stretch sensory nerve endings. Can be due to inflammation, obstruction, etc. Examples are inflammation of the intestines, stone obstruction of a bile duct or within the kidney.

**Colitis**   *Quick Reference:* Inflammation of the colon.

*Advanced Reference:* Usually the large bowel. Common causes are bacterial food poisoning and various types of dysentery.

**Collagen**   *Quick Reference:* An insoluble protein.

*Advanced Reference:* A group of proteins of which the molecules form long fibres. The principal fibrous component of connective tissue. Many body components are regularly broken down and re-synthesised but when collagen is degraded there is little regeneration. This is why ageing is said to be a condition of connective tissue.

**Collateral**   *Quick Reference:* Alternative route for blood flow.

*Advanced Reference:* Refers to blood supply which develops as an alternative route when the main arterial system is interrupted and involves the enlargement and activation of smaller networks.

**Colles fracture**   *Quick Reference:* Fracture of the wrist.

*Advanced Reference:* Usually due to a fall on the palm of the hand forcing back the wrist. Consequently, the radius is broken off and displaced backwards. Due to the connection between the *radius* and *ulna* bones, there is commonly injury to the latter or adjoining ligaments.

**Colloid**   *Quick Reference:* A suspension of particles rather than an actual solution.

*Advanced Reference:* The term is used to indicate a group of IV solutions containing large molecules which determine them to remain in the circulation as they cannot pass through the vessel walls (semipermeable membrane) and exert osmotic pressure that draws fluid into the vessels from the surrounding tissues. This is the function of plasma expanders such as *dextran, haemaccel*, etc.

**Colon**   *Quick Reference:* The main part of the large intestine.

*Advanced Reference:* Begins in the right iliac fossa, where the small intestine joins the caecum at the illeo-caecal junction. This is followed by the ascending colon, transverse colon and descending colon which become the sigmoid colon and terminates at the rectum.

**Colostomy**   *Quick Reference:* A surgical procedure to form a temporary or permanent opening onto the surface of the abdomen.

*Advanced Reference:* A colostomy takes over the natural function of the rectum. It is performed when there is an obstruction in the large intestine. The intestinal contents are collected into a colostomy bag.

**Colporrhaphy**   *Quick Reference:* (col-pora-fi) Surgical repair of the vagina.

*Advanced Reference:* There are two procedures, namely anterior and posterior. Anterior involves prolapse of the bladder into the vagina (cystocele), usually following childbirth and posterior, which involves prolapse of the rectum into the vagina (rectocele).

C

**Colposcopy**   *Quick Reference:* Performed for patients with an abnormal pap smear suggestive of dysplasia.

*Advanced Reference:* A diagnostic examination to identify abnormal cells in the vulva, vagina or cervix such as dysplasia and carcinoma *in situ*.

**Coma**   *Quick Reference:* A state of deep unconsciousness.

*Advanced Reference:* Deep unconsciousness in which the patient cannot be roused, all reflexes such as coughing and blinking are totally absent. Also the patient has no response to painful stimuli.

**Commensal**   *Quick Reference:* An organism that lives in or on another species.

*Advanced Reference:* This organism can live in harmony within or on the body without causing any ill effects.

**Common bile duct**   *Quick Reference:* A duct that conveys bile from the gall bladder to the duodenum.

*Advanced Reference:* Can become blocked with gallstones requiring **cholecystectomy** (open surgery, **laparoscopic** removal or shock-wave therapy).

**Compliance**   *Quick Reference:* Indicates the degree of stiffness of the lungs.

*Advanced Reference:* Also involves the elasticity and distensibility of the chest wall as well as a number of related factors, i.e. respiratory disease, anatomical anomalies, etc. A decrease in compliance results in the need for a greater effort during respiration. If the lungs inflate easily they are said to have a high compliance. Therefore, a low compliance indicates difficult inflation.

**Concussion**   *Quick Reference:* Shaking of the brain, caused by a blow to the head causing temporary loss of consciousness.

*Advanced Reference:* Any damage to the head can cause the brain to violently shake within the skull. This then causes damage to the brain and the tissues become bruised. The result causes loss of consciousness and concussion.

**Conduction anaesthesia**   *Quick Reference:* Alternative term indicating regional anaesthesia.

*Advanced Reference:* Indicates drugs that act locally to block nerve impulses before they reach the *CNS*.

**Congenital**   *Quick Reference:* Means 'present at birth'.

*Advanced Reference:* Present from birth but not necessarily hereditary.

**Conjunctiva**   *Quick Reference:* A transparent covering of the eyeball.

*Advanced Reference:* A delicate membrane covering the inside of the eyelids and the front of the eye.

**Consent**   *Quick Reference:* To give permission.

*Advanced Reference:* An important part of the pre-operative process involving the patient giving their permission for treatment to take place.

Consent can be expressed in writing or verbally or given on behalf by a guardian or a legally appointed person.

**Continuous suture**   *Quick Reference:* Suturing technique.

*Advanced Reference:* Consists of a series of stitches, of which only the first and last are tied as opposed to an interrupted suture when each throw through the skin is knotted. Continuous technique is not widely favoured because a break at any point may mean a disruption of the entire suture line.

**Contraception**   *Quick Reference:* Birth control to prevent a pregnancy.

*Advanced Reference:* Artificial prevention of a pregnancy by using various methods of birth control.

**Controlled drugs**   *Quick Reference:* Term used in relation to medications that are controlled under law.

*Advanced Reference:* A number of evolving laws (Dangerous Drugs Act, Controlled Drugs, Misuse of Drugs Act, etc.) have overseen the control, use and handling of certain classified drugs.

**Contusion**   *Quick Reference:* A bruise.

*Advanced Reference:* Injury to deep tissue through intact skin.

**Convulsion**   *Quick Reference:* A fit or seizure.

*Advanced Reference:* Involuntary, spasmodic muscular contractions. Can be seen in patients with epilepsy or head injuries.

**Co-proxamol**   *Quick Reference:* A compound analgesic.

*Advanced Reference:* It is a combination of the narcotic dextropropoxyphene with paracetamol.

**Cornea**   *Quick Reference:* Transparent part of the eyeball.

*Advanced Reference:* The cornea lies over the pupil and iris through which we see. If it becomes scarred by injury or disease, vision is disturbed or lost.

**Coronary arteries**   *Quick Reference:* Arteries which supply the heart muscle itself.

*Advanced Reference:* The right and left coronary arteries branch off the aorta as it leaves the heart. The left divides into an anterior interventricular branch which passes downwards between the ventricles to the apex of the heart and a left circumflex branch which runs round between the left atrium and ventricle. The right coronary artery runs round between the right atrium and ventricle, and supplies the right ventricle and the sino-atrial node.

**Corpuscle**   *Quick Reference:* Small body or cell.

*Advanced Reference:* Generally used to describe the red blood cells.

**Corrugated tubing**   *Quick Reference:* Refers to the design of tubing used in patients' anaesthetic and ventilator circuits.

*Advanced Reference:* Originally referred to black rubber corrugated tubing but now also includes plastic clear varieties. So designed to allow for stretching, collection of vapour in exhaled breath while allowing for increased tubing diameter.

**Cortex**   *Quick Reference:* The outer layer.

*Advanced Reference:* The outer layer of an organ or other structures such as bone, brain, kidney and adrenal gland.

**Corticosteroids**   *Quick Reference:* Steroid hormones.

*Advanced Reference:* Produced and secreted by the cortex of the adrenal glands or produced synthetically. Best known is hydrocortisone which is used primarily as an anti-inflammatory.

**COSHH**   *Quick Reference:* Control of substances hazardous to health.

*Advanced Reference:* An act brought out under the Health and Safety (H&S) Act, which concentrates on the control and use of substances in the workplace which may be harmful to health if used without assessment and control. The COSHH Act has been constantly updated since first being introduced in the late 1980s. In relation to hospitals may involve cleaning and sterilising fluids, gases, vapours and even the reconstitution of medicines, etc.

**CPAP**   *Quick Reference:* Continuous positive airway pressure

*Advanced Reference:* Indicates the application of positive airway pressure throughout all phases of spontaneous ventilation. Designed to reduce airway collapse and so increase arterial oxygenation.

**CPR**   *Quick Reference:* Cardiopulmonary resuscitation.

*Advanced Reference:* Involves supplying artificial ventilation of the lungs and chest/heart compressions for a patient who has ceased breathing and has no cardiac output.

**Cremophor**   *Quick Reference:* Solubilising (emulsifying) agent used in drug preparations.

*Advanced Reference:* The use of cremophor was highlighted when suspected of being responsible for some of the adverse effects of the now withdrawn induction agent, althesin.

**Crepitus**   *Quick Reference:* Grating noise or sensation.

*Advanced Reference:* Crackling sound heard with a ***stethoscope*** over inflamed lungs or the sounds made by broken bones moving against each other.

**Cricoid  cartilage**   *Quick  Reference:* The  uppermost  ring  of  cartilage around the ***trachea***.

*Advanced Reference:* Ring-shaped cartilage at the lower end of the larynx. It forms the only complete ring within the trachea, all others being C-shaped, with the space towards the rear intended to facilitate the oesophagus.

**Cricothyrotomy**  *Quick Reference:* Emergency access to the upper respiratory tract.

*Advanced Reference:* An emergency procedure where access is gained to the respiratory tract via the cricothyroid membrane using a variety of devices, usually because of upper airway obstruction.

**Critical care**  *Quick Reference:* Refers to specific areas and departments of hospitals.

*Advanced Reference:* Term used commonly to indicate areas involved in emergency and critical care of patients, e.g. accident and emergency (A&E), intensive therapy unit (*ITU*), operating theatres.

**Critical incidents**  *Quick Reference:* Indicates an event or set of events/actions that are considered of such serious nature that they must be highlighted and formally reported upon.

*Advanced Reference:* An increasingly used process in theatres where once common and almost taken for granted occurences are now formally investigated, reflected and fed back on in an attempt to bring about change, improvement or instigate further action. Due mainly to increased professional accountability and litigation and may involve staff, processes or equipment.

**Crohn's disease**  *Quick Reference:* (crones) An inflammatory condition of the digestive tract.

*Advanced Reference:* Can affect anywhere throughout the digestive tract. The symptoms may mimic acute appendicitis with chronic diarrhoea and loss of weight.

**Cross matching**  *Quick Reference:* Refers to establishing the compatibility of a patient's blood, cross-match (X-match).

*Advanced Reference:* Involves identifying a patient's blood group when blood replacement is considered necessary.

**Croup**  *Quick Reference:* A harsh cough and strained noisy breathing in children.

*Advanced Reference:* Causes vary from retarded growth of the larynx to allergy and both viral and bacterial infections.

**Cruciate**  *Quick Reference:* (crushe-e-ate) Anterior and posterior ligament in the knee.

*Advanced Reference:* Gives stability to the knee. The cruciate ligament limits forward movement of the tibia on the femur and is often ruptured in sporting activities by a sharp twisting movement.

**Crush syndrome**   *Quick Reference:* Condition brought on following trauma.
*Advanced Reference:* Involves the trapping of a limb and the consequent impairment of the circulation. There is a build-up of toxins, i.e. histamine, lactic acid, carbon dioxide and when the limb is released, these enter the general circulation causing toxic shock. The time a limb is trapped for is critical in terms of release and availability of advanced care. Some protocols cite that if a limb, etc. has been trapped for 10 min, no attempt at removal should be made until advanced help arrives, whereas others state 30 min.

**Cryo (surgery)**   *Quick Reference:* (crio) Destruction of tissue by freezing.
*Advanced Reference:* Cryo is from the Greek meaning cold. Involves a number of agents, e.g. liquid nitrogen, nitrous oxide. Used in *ophthalmics*, *dermatology*, *urology*, etc.

**Crystalloid**   *Quick Reference:* (cris-tall-oid) Refers to clear IV solutions.
*Advanced Reference:* More correctly, refers to solutions which may pass through a semipermeable membrane as opposed to the osmotic action of *colloids* which are solutions containing large molecules.

**Crystapen**   *Quick Reference:* (cris-ta-pen) A proprietary antibiotic.
*Advanced Reference:* Used to treat many forms of infection and prevent rheumatic fever.

**CSF**   *Quick Reference:* Cerebrospinal fluid.
*Advanced Reference:* The fluid in which the CNS lies, contained by the meninges, which are the covering membranes.

**CSSD**   *Quick Reference:* Central Sterile Services Department.
*Advanced Reference:* At one time a hospital-based sterilising and supply department. In more recent times these departments have given way to district, regional or private organisations. Some theatres however, still maintain a Theatre Sterile Services Department (TSSU).

**Culture**   *Quick Reference:* The growing of micro-organisms or cells.
*Advanced Reference:* The process of growing micro-organisms or other living cells in artificial circumstances on suitable materials, such as *agar* mixed with blood or broth. A *culture swab*, also known as swab-stick, is used for bacteriology specimens (pus, etc.)

**Cut down**   *Quick Reference:* To make access to a blood vessel via incision through the skin and underlying tissues.
*Advanced Reference:* Procedure used when venous access is not possible via direct *cannulation*, usually due to peripheral vascular shutdown.

**Cutting needle**   *Quick Reference:* Type of suturing needle.
*Advanced Reference:* A cutting needle is triangular in cross section and has its cutting edge directed towards the wound and its flat surface

away from the wound. Used for suturing tough or dense tissue, e.g. fascia and skin.

**CVP**   *Quick Reference:* Central venous pressure.

*Advanced Reference:* Refers to the pressure created by the circulating blood volume. Measured in $H_2Ocm$ with a manometer or transducer from a catheter inserted through a central vein and sited just outside of the right atrium.

**Cyanosis**   *Quick Reference:* (sigh-a-nosis) Blue tinge of the skin and *mucous membranes.*

*Advanced Reference:* Caused by insufficient oxygenation of the blood.

**Cyclimorph**   *Quick Reference:* (sike-la-morf) Proprietary form of *morphine* combined with *cyclizine.*

*Advanced Reference:* The combination of narcotic analgesic, *anti-emetic* and *antihistamine,* used to treat moderate to severe pain.

**Cyclizine**   *Quick Reference:* (cike-la-zine) An antihistamine and anti-emetic.

*Advanced Reference:* Used in the treatment of motion sickness and general nausea and vomiting.

**Cyclopropane**   *Quick Reference:* (cike-lo-propane) Gas used as an inhalational anaesthetic.

*Advanced Reference:* Now withdrawn from use but was used for both induction and maintenance of anaesthesia. However, had the disadvantage of being highly explosive and wherever possible was avoided where ignition was possible, e.g. when diathermy was in use.

**Cyclosporin**   *Quick Reference:* A powerful immunosuppressant.

*Advanced Reference:* Particularly used to limit tissue rejection during transplant surgery. A patient on cyclosporin is particularly vulnerable to infection.

**Cyst**   *Quick Reference:* (sist) A hollow swelling usually containing fluid, a bladder.

*Advanced Reference:* Appear most often in the skin and in the ovaries but can develop in many alternative body sites. Cystic means pertaining to a cyst.

**Cystitis**   *Quick Reference:* (sist-it-is) Inflammation of the urinary bladder.

*Advanced Reference:* Usually due to bacterial infection and because of the shorter urethra is more common in women as this allows easier access for ascending infection.

**Cystocele**   *Quick Reference:* (sist-o-seal) Herniation of the bladder into the vagina.

*Advanced Reference:* Due to overstretching of the vagina wall during childbirth.

**Cystoscope**   *Quick Reference:* Instrument for examining the interior of the urinary bladder.

*Advanced Reference:* An endoscopic procedure which involves the passage of a telescope via the urethra into the bladder.

**Cystostomy**   *Quick Reference:* Opening of the bladder to the surface.

*Advanced Reference:* Is a surgical procedure whereby an opening is made into the bladder via the abdominal wall. Usually carried out when normal exit of the bladder is blocked, etc. Cystotomy indicates opening the bladder by surgical incision.

**Cytology**   *Quick Reference:* (sigh-tol-ogy) The study of cells utilising microscopy.

*Advanced Reference:* The study of the function and structure of cells. An example is cervical smear of the cervix.

**Cytotoxics**   *Quick Reference:* Drug used mainly in the treatment of cancer.

*Advanced Reference:* Group of anticancer drugs that have the essential property of preventing normal cell replication and so inhibiting the growth of tumours or excess cells in body fluids.

**Dacron**   *Quick Reference:* Relates to vascular and thoracic surgery grafts.

*Advanced Reference:* Dacron grafts are either of the knitted or woven type. Comprised of polyethylene and is kink resistant and elastic in nature. Some are impregnated with gelatin or collagen, which helps seal the graft. Knitted grafts require pre-clotting with the patient's blood.

**Dacron cuff**   *Quick Reference:* A sheath of dacron surrounding an arterial or venous catheter.

*Advanced Reference:* Designed to adhere to the surrounding tissue and prevent accidental displacement. Found with intravenous (IV) feeding lines and often used in combination with tunnelling of the catheter.

**Damping**   *Quick Reference:* Term related to recording systems indicating a reduction in amplitude (size) and therefore interference of the recording trace, etc.

*Advanced Reference:* Seen in invasive arterial monitoring systems when the trace reading is affected by air bubbles in the system, blood clots or kinking of the manometer tubing.

**D&C**   *Quick Reference:* Dilatation and curettage. A gynaecological procedure.

*Advanced Reference:* Involves dilatation of the os of the cervix and a curette is used to remove endometrium.

**Dantrium**   *Quick Reference:* Proprietary skeletal muscle relaxant, e.g. dantrolene sodium.

*Advanced Reference:* Used in the treatment of ***malignant hyperthermia***. This preparation is in combination with mannitol, which acts as a preservative.

**Dead space**   *Quick Reference:* Area where no gas exchange takes place.

*Advanced Reference:* Anatomical dead space includes the mouth, nose, pharynx and large airways. Equipment dead space involves anaesthetic masks, circuits, etc. Insertion of an endotracheal tube (ET) tube reduces dead space as it bypasses the anatomical dead space. Mask anaesthesia greatly increases dead space. The issue of equipment dead space is of greater importance with paediatric circuits.

**Debridement**   *Quick Reference:* Thorough cleansing of a wound.
*Advanced Reference:* Involves cleaning and removal of foreign material and damaged tissue, usually following *traumatic* injury.

**Decadron**   *Quick Reference:* A proprietary corticosteroid.
*Advanced Reference:* A preparation of dexamethasone used to replace steroid loss and in the treatment of shock.

**Decapitation**   *Quick Reference:* Literally, cutting off of the head.
*Advanced Reference:* Can indicate the head itself above the shoulders/neck or the head of a bone.

**Decapsulation**   *Quick Reference:* (de-cap-su-la-shun) Surgical incision and removal of a fibrous capsule.
*Advanced Reference:* Renal decapsulation is the freeing and removal of the capsule surrounding the kidney.

**Decompression**   *Quick Reference:* To remove internal pressure. Surgical procedure designed to release or relieve pressure on an organ or structure.
*Advanced Reference:* Example would be, drilling or removal of part of the skull to relieve intracranial pressure, removal of bone, etc. pressing on the spinal cord.

**Defence mechanism**   *Quick Reference:* An immunological mechanism by which the body resists invasion by pathogens or harmful organisms.
*Advanced Reference:* Also used to indicate a psychological means of coping with conflict or anxiety.

**Defibrillation**   *Quick Reference:* Applying an electric shock across the heart using a defibrillator.
*Advanced Reference:* An attempt to restore normal rhythm to the heart in ventricular or atrial fibrillation by applying energy in the form of an electric shock. This depolarises the cardiac cells and allows the *sino-atrial* node to take over and restore *sinus rhythm*.

**Defunctioning colostomy**   *Quick Reference:* A surgical intervention for disease of the lower colon and rectum.
*Advanced Reference:* Used where there is a need to either rest the colon following an anastomosis or to have a permanent bypass in order to keep the faeces away from the diseased part. A loop of colon is brought out onto the skin so that the faeces is discharged into a *colostomy* bag attached to the skin.

**Deglove**   *Quick Reference:* Injury to extremities, i.e. fingers, hand, arm, toes, leg, foot.
*Advanced Reference:* Involves the peeling off of tissue down to the bone including neurovascular bundles and possibly tendons, usually due to trauma.

**Dehiscence**   *Quick Reference:* (de-his-ense) Splitting open.
  *Advanced Reference:* Term applied to the breakdown of surgical incisions in the post-operative period. Usually due to infection. Used in relation to the slang term 'burst abdomen'.

**Dehydration**   *Quick Reference:* A reduction in the total water content of the body.
  *Advanced Reference:* Excessive fluid loss may be due to reduced or lack of intake, sweating, persistent vomiting and diarrhoea. Signs and symptoms include thirst, muscle cramp and weakness, low urine output of less than 400 ml/24 h.(*oliguria*).

**Delirium**   *Quick Reference:* Disturbance of the brain, causing confusion, excitement and other symptoms of disorganised mental activity.
  *Advanced Reference:* Due to injury, fever, poisoning, etc.

**Delorme's procedure**   *Quick Reference:* A surgical intervention of the perineal area for repair of a complete full thickness rectal prolapse.
  *Advanced Reference:* A complete prolapse is a full thickness rectal *prolapse* protruding from the anus, contains two layers of the rectal wall. Occurs most commonly in older adults, with females more affected than males and is associated with weak pelvic and anal muscles.

**Deltoid**   *Quick Reference:* Triangular, deltoid muscle.
  *Advanced Reference:* This muscle lies on the ***anterior*** border and upper surface of the outer third of the clavicle and enables the arm to *abduct*, flex and rotate.

**Demand pacemaker**   *Quick Reference:* Device used to stimulate the heart electrically.
  *Advanced Reference:* Used when the heart and impulses are not sufficient. Works by measuring the interval between beats and if the normal value is exceeded the pacemaker delivers a stimulating pulse.

**Dementia**   *Quick Reference:* (dem-en-sha) Loss of intellectual functions.
  *Advanced Reference:* Resulting in deficient memory and concentration. The condition is progressive. Although can also be caused by thyroid disturbance, infection, etc. but most cases are due to the degenerative processes of ageing.

**Dendrite**   *Quick Reference:* Filament of a nerve cell.
  *Advanced Reference:* Carries electrical signals from the synapse to the cell body. Each neurone (nerve cell) has many dendrites.

**Denervate**   *Quick Reference:* (den-er-vate) De-nerve, i.e. to remove nerves.
  *Advanced Reference:* Denervated – without nerve supply. Denervation – removal or severence of the nerve supply. As happens following certain types of surgery, i.e. ***transplantation***.

**Deoxygenate**  *Quick Reference:* (de-ox-a-gen-ate) Deprived of oxygen.
*Advanced Reference:* To become deplete of oxygen. Desaturate.

**Depolarisation**  *Quick Reference:* The neutralisation of an electric charge.
*Advanced Reference:* A depolarising block involves skeletal muscle paralysis associated with the loss of polarity of the motor end plate as occurs following the administration of a cholinergic antagonist.

**Depo-medrone**  *Quick Reference:* Proprietary corticosteroid.
*Advanced Reference:* Used in the treatment of inflammation and to relieve allergic disorders such as rheumatoid arthritis, hay fever and asthma. Is a preparation of the steroid methylprednisolone.

**Dermatology**  *Quick Reference:* The medical speciality dealing with skin diseases.
*Advanced Reference:* The dermis being the connective tissue underlying the epithelium of the skin. A dermatome is an instrument for cutting slices of skin for skin grafting.

**Dermatomes**  *Quick Reference:* The area of skin innervated by the branches of a single spinal nerve.
*Advanced Reference:* Useful with regional anaesthesia in determining the extent of the block as areas of the skin are supplied by particular spinal nerves.

**Dermoid cyst:**  *Quick Reference:* A congenital type of cyst.
*Advanced Reference:* Formed by a collection of cancerous cells that contain one or more of the three primary embryonic layers of skin, hair or teeth.

**Desflurane**  *Quick Reference:* (dez-floor-ane) Volatile anaesthetic agent.
*Advanced Reference:* Requires an elaborate vaporiser which is heated and pressurised. Relatively insoluble so induction and recovery are rapid.

**Detached retina**  *Quick Reference:* Can occur spontaneously or as a result of trauma.
*Advanced Reference:* The retina, or part of it, separates from the choroids. The patient complains of a gradual decline in their field of vision.

**Detergent**  *Quick Reference:* Cleansing agent.
*Advanced Reference:* Detergents work by lowering surface tension which enables water to penetrate better and remove grease by forming an emulsion.

**Detruser**  *Quick Reference:* (det-rus-er) A muscle that has the action of expelling a substance.
*Advanced Reference:* The detrusor muscle in the urinary bladder provides a muscular coat. Dysfunction of this muscle can lead to urinary *incontinence*.

**Dettol**  *Quick Reference:* Antiseptic and disinfectant.
  *Advanced Reference:* Used to treat abrasions and minor wounds as well as disinfecting instruments. It is a preparation of chloroxylenol.

**Dextran**  *Quick Reference:* An IV plasma substitute.
  *Advanced Reference:* A carbohydrate consisting of glucose units. Used as a plasma expander in haemorrhage or shock, such as burns. Can interfere with cross-matching (X-matching) of blood. Two major preparations are namely *Dextran 40*, a 10% solution in glucose or saline and used to improve blood flow in the limbs and preventing thrombosis and *Dextran 70* a 6% concentration in glucose or saline 70 and used to expand blood volume.

**Dextrocardia**  *Quick Reference:* Abnormal position of the heart.
  *Advanced Reference:* Dextrocardia is a rare heart condition, caused by the unusual positioning of the heart which is usually rotated to the right, the patient may not even know of any problems until connected to an electrocardiogram (ECG) for the first time, where an abnormality will show up on the waves representing the heartbeat, the waves will show an inversion of activity, i.e. the P-wave will be completely opposite to its original position, most individuals who are affected by this rare condition (which is present from birth) can lead a normal life.

**Dextrolyte**  *Quick Reference:* (dex-tro-light) Proprietary sodium solution.
  *Advanced Reference:* Used to treat mild to moderate sodium depletion as in dehydration. Produced in an oral preparation containing sodium chloride, potassium chloride, glucose and sodium lactate.

**Dextro-saline**  *Quick Reference:* IV solution.
  *Advanced Reference:* A mixture of 0.18% saline and 4.3% dextrose. This equates to 0.18 g of sodium and 4.3 g dextrose per 100 ml.

**DF118**  *Quick Reference:* Proprietary narcotic analgesic.
  *Advanced Reference:* Used to treat moderate to severe pain. Available as tablets and elixir as well as in ampoules for injection as a controlled drug. A preparation of dihydrocodeine tartrate.

**Diabetes**  *Quick Reference:* A somewhat general term but characterised by excessive urine excretion (*polyuria*).
  *Advanced Reference: Diabetes insipidus* is a rare form in which the kidney tubules do not reabsorb sufficient water. This can be due to inadequate production of antidiuretic hormone (**ADH**) production by the pituitary gland leading to excessive production of dilute urine, a defective collecting duct or the ADH receptors of the renal tubules being defective. *Diabetes mellitus* involves a relative or absolute lack of insulin due to deficiency of its secretion from the pancreas. This can in turn lead to uncontrolled carbohydrate metabolism. Signs and symptoms of diabetes mellitus are lassitude and debility, loss of weight, pruritis and a lowered resistance to infection.

**Diagnosis**   *Quick Reference:* The determination of the nature of a disease.

*Advanced Reference:* Diagnosis refers to something that is used to determine the cause of an illness or disorder. Differential diagnosis distinguishes between conditions with similar symptoms. Signs & symptoms, i.e. signs are something that may be observed in the process of diagnosis whereas symptoms occur as the result of an illness and are usually recognised by the patient causing them to seek medical help.

**Dialysis**   *Quick Reference:* (die-al-a-sis) To separate, filter.

*Advanced Reference:* Selective diffusion through a membrane. As applied in the artificial kidney machine where a membrane divides a stream of the patient's blood, taken from an artery and returned through a vein, from a prepared solution of salts, glucose, etc., which is in the same concentration (*isotonic*) as normal blood.

**Diaphragm**   *Quick Reference:* (di-a-fram) Sheet of muscle separating the *thorax* from the abdomen.

*Advanced Reference:* The diaphragm arises from the lumbar vertebrae, the lower ribs and the lower end of the *sternum*. It converges on a flat sheet of dense fibrous tissue and the whole structure forms a sort of dome. A diaphragmatic hernia is a protrusion of a part of the stomach through the oesophageal opening in the diaphragm.

**Diaphysis**   *Quick Reference:* The shaft of a long bone.

*Advanced Reference:* Consists of compact bone enclosing the medullary cavity.

**Diastole**   *Quick Reference:* Resting phase of the heart.

*Advanced Reference:* Diastole precedes the systole phase and indicates the period when the ventricles are filling with blood.

**Diathermy**   *Quick Reference:* (di-ah-ther-me) A high-frequency alternating current (AC) which produces heat.

*Advanced Reference:* The heat is generated not by the electric current but is due to oscillation of the ions in the tissues. A pulsed high-frequency AC coagulates the tissues with minimal disruption whereas a blended current of cutting and coagulation improves haemostasis. Monopolar diathermy is most commonly used in the operating room and consists of the electrosurgical generator, active electrode, patient return electrode and the patient. Bipolar diathermy does not require an earthing plate. The circuit consists of the generator, coaxial lead from the instrument and the patient which carries and returns the current. The earthing, or more accurately the return electrode, forms an important component of the whole unit and if improperly applied can lead to burns. It should be positioned on a well-vascularised area, as close to the operating site as possible, away from bony prominences and any prosthesis as this could interfere with conductivity.

**Diazemuls**   *Quick Reference:* Proprietary anxiolytic drug.
*Advanced Reference:* Used to treat anxiety and to provide sedation for minor surgery. Also used as a premedication as it also has some skeletal muscle-relaxant properties. Produced as an emulsion for injection. Is a preparation of the *benzodiazepine*, diazepam.

**DIC**   *Quick Reference:* Disseminated intravascular clotting.
*Advanced Reference:* Associated with many conditions, e.g. severe haemorrhage, pancreatitis, major surgery and cardiopulmonary bypass. Abnormal coagulation occurs within the micro-circulation using up clotting factors and reducing peripheral flow. This results in reduced clotting efficiency and profuse bleeding. Treatment is with heparin as it prevents further using up of coagulation factors permitting normal clotting function.

**Dicrotic notch**   *Quick Reference:* A double beat.
*Advanced Reference:* Is when an artery expands a second time giving rise to a dicrotic beat (notch) as seen on an invasive arterial monitoring trace. Happens when the output from the heart is forceful and the tension of the pulse is low.

**Diethyl ether**   *Quick Reference:* (die-eth-al) A general anaesthetic (GA) agent.
*Advanced Reference:* Anaesthetic ether. Is flammable and explosive in the presence of oxygen. Causes nausea, vomiting.

**Diffuse**   *Quick Reference:* Scattered or widespread.
*Advanced Reference:* The opposite to diffuse being localised.

**Diffusion**   *Quick Reference:* Spontaneous movement of molecules in a liquid or gas.
*Advanced Reference:* The distribution leads to an equalising out with the intention of reaching a uniform concentration. As with gas exchange in the lungs between oxygen and carbon dioxide.

**Digestion**   *Quick Reference:* The process of breaking down food in the stomach and intestines.
*Advanced Reference:* The food is broken down into soluble and diffusible products capable of being absorbed by the blood.

**Digoxin**   *Quick Reference:* Heart stimulant.
*Advanced Reference:* Derived from the *Digitalis* plant. Regulates and strengthens heartbeat.

**Dilatation**   *Quick Reference:* The process of stretching a constricted passage.
*Advanced Reference:* Strictures occur in the urethra which have to be dilated. Anal dilatation involves stretching of the muscle fibres. There are numerous dilators, specific to their intended use.

**Diltiazem**   *Quick Reference:* Vasodilator and *calcium antagonist* drug, e.g. tildiem.

*Advanced Reference:* Used in the prevention and treatment of angina pectoris, especially when beta-blockers have not been effective.

**Dioxin**   *Quick Reference:* An organic chemical compound.
*Advanced Reference:* It is **carcinogenic** and can cause genetic changes leading to congenital deformities. The incomplete or inefficient burning of plastics (polyvinyl chloride, PVC) in hospital incinerators was highlighted as a likely source. Also referred to as agent orange, a defoliant used in wartime.

**Diprivan**   *Quick Reference:* Anaesthetic-induction agent.
*Advanced Reference:* Proprietary form of propofol. Also used as a maintenance agent. Has a rapid recovery and fast excretion time so is recommended for day-case surgery.

**Disarticulation**   *Quick Reference:* Amputation or separation at a joint.
*Advanced Reference:* An example is disarticulation of the leg, separated at the hip joint. Sometimes referred to as hind-quarter.

**Disc**   *Quick Reference:* A flattened circular structure.
*Advanced Reference:* Intervertebral disc is a fibrous-cartilaginous pad that separates the bodies of the two adjacent vertebrae. Discectomy is excision of part or whole of an intervertebal disc. The optic disc is a white spot in the retina where the optic nerve enters.

**Discard-a-pad**   *Quick Reference:* Pad used by the scrub practitioner to safely dispose of sharps.
*Advanced Reference:* Besides being used for the disposal of needles, sutures, blades, etc. can also be an aid to efficient checking of the needles.

**Disinfectant**   *Quick Reference:* (dis-in-fek-tant) Surface cleaning fluid.
*Advanced Reference:* An agent that disinfects; applied particularly to agents used on inanimate objects; whereas an antiseptic, is an agent that is capable of destroying *micro-organisms.* Can be known as an antiseptic, i.e. *antiseptic **betadine*** a skin preparation used at the beginning of operations to clean the skin.

**Dislocation**   *Quick Reference:* (dis-lo-ka-shun) In Latin locare means place. Is a popular term that indicates moving out of position.
*Advanced Reference:* The displacement of any part, more especially of a bone from its natural position upon another at a joint, e.g. dislocated hip.

**Dissect**   *Quick Reference:* (di-sekt ) To cut carefully in the study of anatomy.
*Advanced Reference:* During an operation to separate according to natural lines of structure.

**Dissecting forceps**   *Quick Reference:* A surgical instrument used for holding tissues.

*Advanced Reference:* Dissecting forceps come in many shapes and sizes and are used for holding tissues. They can be toothed or non-toothed. Some of the most common in use being Adsons, Lanes, McIndoe, Gillies, Debakey and Bonnies, etc.

**Distal**   *Quick Reference:* (dis-tal) Further from central.

*Advanced Reference:* Remote; farther from any point of reference; opposite to *proximal*. In dentistry used to designate a position on the dental arch farther from the median line of the jaw. Situated away from the centre of the body or point of origin.

**Distention**   *Quick Reference:* (dis-ten-shun) Enlargement.

*Advanced Reference:* Abdominal distention is the result of swelling as a result of gas in the intestines or fluid in the abdominal cavity.

**Diuresis**   *Quick Reference:* (di-u-re-sis) More urine than normal.

*Advanced Reference:* Increased excretion of urine.

**Diuretic**   *Quick Reference:* (die-your-etic) Drug or substance which increases the flow of urine.

*Advanced Reference:* Diuretics act on either the distal tubule and others that act on the loop of Henle, and these are termed loop diuretics, a common example being frusemide (lasix). Mannitol also causes an increase of urine output but due to the action of osmotic pressure.

**Diverticulitis**   *Quick Reference:* (di-ver-tik-u-li-tis) Colon inflammation.

*Advanced Reference:* Inflammation of the diverticulum especially refers to inflammation relating to colonic diverticula. Usually present with lower abdominal pain, colic and constipation may occur and intestinal obstruction or absences may develop. *Inflammation* of *Meckal's diverticulum* may produce symptoms similar to appendicitis.

**Division of adhesions**   *Quick Reference:* The surgical separating of fibrous bands or structures to which organs and various anatomy have adhered.

*Advanced Reference:* Usually occur following previous surgery and can cause internal obstruction.

**Documents**   *Quick Reference:* Refers to patients' case-files, etc. and any related correspondence, results of investigations, etc.

*Advanced Reference:* An original or official paper relied upon as a basis, proof or support of something; a writing (such as a care pathway, care plan, theatre pathway) conveying information; a legal document that may be required as evidence in a court of law.

**Donor**   *Quick Reference:* (do-nor) One who gives his blood or his own organs, e.g. a kidney, or tissue to another who is histocompatible.

*Advanced Reference:* Universal donor – someone who has group O (negative) blood.

**Dopamine**   *Quick Reference:* A neurotransmitter and sympathomimetic, e.g. intropin.

*Advanced Reference:* Used to treat cardiogenic shock following heart attack or during surgery. Sometimes used in small doses to dilate the renal artery following kidney transplantation.

**Doppler**   *Quick Reference:* A machine that works by relating the drop in pitch of a note when a moving source of sound passes the recording source.

*Advanced Reference:* Doppler is used to detect flow in blood vessels, i.e. for central venous pressure (CVP) insertion, etc. with the use of a surface probe.

**Dopram**   *Quick Reference:* Proprietary preparation of doxapram.

*Advanced Reference:* A respiratory stimulant used to relieve severe respiratory difficulties such as post-operative respiratory depression. Side effects include a rise in blood pressure (BP) and heart rate, and dizziness.

**Dorsalis pedis**   *Quick Reference:* Refers to the artery in the upper foot above the toes.

*Advanced Reference:* Used to take a pulse and is palpable between the first and second metatarsal bones on top of the foot. Sometimes used as a site for arterial cannulation.

**Dorsiflexion**   *Quick Reference:* Bending backwards of the fingers or toes.

*Advanced Reference:* Indicates bending backwards but in many cases actually upwards, e.g. the great toe.

**Dorsum**   *Quick Reference:* The back or posterior surfaces.

*Advanced Reference:* Example is, the back of the hand. Dorsal relates to the back or posterior of an organ.

**Dosimetry**   *Quick Reference:* Giving a dose or measure.

*Advanced Reference:* Involves the determination of the amount, rate and distribution of radiation to be delivered.

**Double-glove**   *Quick Reference:* To don two pairs of gloves to give extra protection for the patient.

*Advanced Reference:* Used regularly in orthopaedic surgery where bone infection is always a possibility and difficult to treat. Can also be used to provide extra protection for the practitioner.

**Draffin suspension rods**   *Quick Reference:* Surgical instrument used during tonsillectomy or surgery of the mouth.

*Advanced Reference:* Made of stainless steel and place in a holder on either side of the patient's head. The tongue plate of the mouth gag fits into the rings on the rods allowing the mouth to stay open and freeing up both hands of the operating surgeon.

**Drain**   *Quick Reference:* A device used in surgery for draining fluid, pus, etc. from a cavity or the operation site.

*Advanced Reference:* Used to drain fluid away from the operative site in the immediate post-operative period. Drains come in two classifications passive and active.

**Drape**   *Quick Reference:* Refers to sterile covering used to cover the operative site.

*Advanced Reference:* Drapes are manufactured from paper or fabric and come in various sizes and shapes to suit the type of surgery being performed.

**Dressings**   *Quick Reference:* A sterile covering placed over a wound after surgery.

*Advanced Reference:* A dressing is applied to protect the wound and act as a visual barrier in the post-operative period.

**Drip**   *Quick Reference:* Slang term used to denote an IV infusion.

*Advanced Reference:* Although at times intended to make reference to the fluid itself, generally indicates the complete drip configuration of IV fluid bag and *giving-set*. A drip stand is basically a pole, which attaches to the table or trolley, or mobile on wheels and designed to hold the IV bag at varying heights.

**Dromoran**   *Quick Reference:* Narcotic analgesic.

*Advanced Reference:* A preparation of the opiate and narcotic levorphanol tartrate. Used to relieve severe pain and enhance GA.

**Droperidol**   *Quick Reference:* Powerful tranquilliser, e.g. droleptan.

*Advanced Reference:* Used in conjunction with *fentanyl* in *neuroleptic* techniques and as an *anti-emetic*. No longer widely used or available in the UK.

**Dual block**   *Quick Reference:* Also known as Phase II block.

*Advanced Reference:* If depolarising agents are given repeatedly, the nature of the block eventually changes and increasingly shows the properties of a non-depolariser making it possible for an *anticholinesterase* to bring about a degree of reversal. If intermittent *suxemethonium infusion* is being used, the recommendation is to allow the block to wear off at intervals.

**Duct**   *Quick Reference:* A tube or channel.

*Advanced Reference:* A channel with well-defined walls for the passage of excretions or secretions.

**Duodenum**   *Quick Reference:* The first part of the intestine.

*Advanced Reference:* The duodenum lies between the stomach and the *jejunum* and measures approximately 20–25 cm in length. The pancreatic and *common bile ducts* open into it.

**Dupuytren's**   *Quick Reference:* (dupe-ya-trons) Painless thickening of the connective tissue of the palm.

*Advanced Reference:* Involves the palmer fascia and the contracture can cause permanent bending and fixation of one or more fingers. Can be due to many causes including trauma. Surgical correction involves a palmer *fasciectomy*.

**Dura**   *Quick Reference:* The dura mater.
*Advanced Reference:* The outermost and toughest of the three meningeal membranes which surround the brain and spinal cord.

**DVT**   *Quick Reference:* Deep vein thrombosis. Formation of a thrombus (blood clot) in the veins, e.g. the inner thigh or lower leg.
*Advanced Reference:* Becomes dangerous if and when the clot breaks free and travels (embolus) through the circulatory system to the lung. Many measures are utilised to help prevent DVT formation, i.e. heparin, heel pad, support stockings, etc.

**Dynamic hip screw**   *Quick Reference:* DHS, a metal internal fixation device used to stabilise certain proximal fractures of the femur.
*Advanced Reference:* Designed to provide strong and stable internal fixation for a variety of fractures of the neck of femur.

**Dynamo**   *Quick Reference:* Power or strength.
*Advanced Reference:* Commonly, a device that generates electricity.

**Dys**   *Quick Reference:* (dis) Prefix indicating 'bad'.
*Advanced Reference:* In medical terms the implied sense is 'difficult'.

**Dysphagia**   *Quick Reference:* (dis-fay-gea) Difficulty in swallowing.
*Advanced Reference:* Can be a symptom of blockage or muscle spasm of the oesophagus.

**Dyspnoea**   *Quick Reference:* (dis-p-nea) Difficulty in breathing.
*Advanced Reference:* Undue shortness of breath or laboured breathing.

**Dysrhythmia**   *Quick Reference:* (dis-rith-mia) Abnormal heart rhythm.
*Advanced Reference:* Term used to indicate disordered or disorganised heart rhythms.

# E

**ECG**   *Quick Reference:* Electrocardiograph.

*Advanced Reference:* A recording or visual display of the electrical changes in the heart muscle taken through electrodes attached to the external chest wall. During routine anaesthesia three leads are applied however patients with heart conditions may require a 12 lead ECG tracing, 12 lead offers a more in depth look at the health status of the heart.

**Echocardiography**   *Quick Reference:* (car-dee-og-raffy) Cardiac imaging using ultrasound.

*Advanced Reference:* The use of ultrasound to examine the heart in terms of both anatomy and function.

**Eclampsia**   *Quick Reference:* (e-clamp-cia) Convulsions during pregnancy due to *toxaemia*.

*Advanced Reference:* Pre-eclampsia is the state preceding the crisis. Eclampsia produces fits/*convulsions* and possible *coma* and is characterised by *oedema, hypertension* and protein in the *urine (proteinuria)*. Immediate treatment is to deliver the baby, as the condition can be fatal to both mother and foetus.

**ECT**   *Quick Reference:* Electro-convulsive therapy.

*Advanced Reference:* Treatment of mental illness by applying a small electric shock to the external scalp with electrodes. This passes through the frontal lobes of the brain and brings about a brief period of unconsciousness followed by convulsion. It is used in the treatment of depression and schizophrenia which do not respond to other treatment regimes.

**-ectomy**   *Quick Reference:* Surgical removal of a part or all of an organ.

*Advanced Reference:* A suffix which describes that an organ or part thereof has been surgically removed/excised, e.g. *appendicectomy*, surgical removal of the appendix.

**Ectopic**   *Quick Reference:* Outside or away from the normal site.

*Advanced Reference:* Ectopic indicates an abnormal anatomical situation or position. Examples being *ectopic pregnancy* (when a fertilised ovum settles and starts to develop in the fallopian tube instead of progressing to the uterus) and also *ectopic heartbeat* (when extra beats originate from an area other than the normal conduction system).

**Ectropian**   *Quick Reference:* Eyelid turned outwards.
*Advanced Reference:* The margin of the eyelid is averted and requires surgery to shorten the lower eyelid. Most commonly seen in the elderly, people with nerve *palsy* or if the skin of the lower eyelid has been scarred following *trauma* or previous surgery.

**Edinburgh Tray System**   *Quick Reference:* A system for surgical tray layout.
*Advanced Reference:* During processing of surgical instruments and in surgical use the adoption of the Edinburgh Tray System is highly effective in locating instruments. The system uses a rolled up length of sterile paper placed beneath the handles of the surgical instruments. The instruments were grouped together without a sterile retaining pin. The systematic order allowed easy access and accountability of the instruments.

**Edrophonium**   *Quick Reference:* (ed-ro-fone-eum) An *anticholinesterase*.
*Advanced Reference:* Available as tensilon.

**EEG**   *Quick Reference:* Electroencephalogram.
*Advanced Reference:* A record of the electrical activity in the brain through electrodes attached to the scalp.

**Efcortisol**   *Quick Reference:* Proprietary preparation of hydrocortisone.
*Advanced Reference:* A corticosteroid used as an anti-inflammatory for allergy, to treat shock and make up a deficiency of steroid hormone.

**Efferent**   *Quick Reference:* Leading away from the centre to the periphery.
*Advanced Reference:* Efferent arterioles/artery exits in the glomerulus of the kidney after entering as the afferent vessel. *Efferent* motor nerves leave the brain to supply the muscles.

**Effusion**   *Quick Reference:* An outpouring of fluid into the tissues or a cavity.
*Advanced Reference:* Examples where this is common are the knee and pleural space and can involve blood serum, etc. Causes can be due to inflammation or congestion.

**Elastic stockings**   *Quick Reference:* Support devices for the legs.
*Advanced Reference:* Used in cases of varicose veins or *oedema* of the legs. Made with various degrees of elasticity according to the support needed. In relation to theatres, are used to prevent deep vein thrombosis (*DVT*) during surgery.

**Elective**   *Quick Reference:* Chosen. Used with reference to type of admission to hospital.
*Advanced Reference:* Used to differentiate between a scheduled and emergency procedure. Common example is an elective Caesarean section as opposed to emergency due to either maternal or foetal complications.

**Electrode**   *Quick Reference:* A conductive point of delivery or return of an electrical charge.

*Advanced Reference:* Electrodes are commonly referred to within the theatre as the stick dots for applying a 3-lead *ECG* to the patient's chest wall. Each electrode provides a connection between the patient and the machine interpreting the electrical activity of the heart. Further examples of electrodes include those used for *EEG*, *ECT* and the grounding plate for *diathermy* is sometimes referred to as an electrode.

**Electrolysis**   *Quick Reference:* (elec-trol-a-sis) Chemical changes brought about by means of electricity. Also refers to a process involving hair removal.

*Advanced Reference:* An example is the passing of electricity through water which decomposes/separates into oxygen and hydrogen.

**Electrolyte**   *Quick Reference:* (elec-tro-lite) A solution which is capable of conducting electricity. A substance that forms a solution through which an electric current can be passed because the molecules involved separate into ions, i.e. groups of atoms with an electrical charge; the cations being attracted to the negative electrode and the anions to the positive.

*Advanced Reference:* Ions are formed when a compound disassociates in a solution, e.g. $NaCl > Na^+ + Cl^-$. The most common being *sodium*, *potassium*, *calcium*, *magnesium*. The resultant solutions have the ability to conduct electricity, hence the term, electrolyte.

**Electromagnetic**   *Quick Reference:* Pertaining to magnetism that is induced by an electric current.

*Advanced Reference:* Involves radiation such as microwaves, X-rays, radio waves, etc.

**Emaciation**   *Quick Reference:* (em-ace-ea-shun) Indicates extreme wasting of body tissues.

*Advanced Reference:* Extreme loss of body weight. Malnourishment. Seen in patients suffering chronic disease and elderly patients admitted for surgery who are deplete in fluids and nourishment.

**Embolism**   *Quick Reference:* (em-bo-lisem) Blocking of a blood vessel by material carried in the bloodstream and can lead to blockage elsewhere within the vascular system, i.e. pulmonary embolism.

*Advanced Reference:* The material (embolus) can be a blood clot, fat, air and less commonly amniotic fluid, fragment from catheter, etc. Removal is termed an embolectomy, usually carried out with a long catheter inserted into the vessel which has an inflatable balloon designed to pass the obstruction in the deflated position, then inflated with saline for extraction.

**EMD**   *Quick Reference:* Electromechanical dissociation, also termed *pulseless electrical activity* (PEA).

*Advanced Reference:* Absence of sufficient cardiac output but displaying (near) normal electrical activity on the *ECG*. Can be due to pulmonary embolism, pneumothorax, hypovolaemia, hypercarbia, etc.

**Emesis**   *Quick Reference:* (em-ee-sis) Medical term for vomiting.
*Advanced Reference:* Emesis can be coupled within further medical terminology, such as *haematemesis*. Relating to the vomiting of blood. An emetic is any substance that can induce vomiting. An *anti-emetic* is a drug administered to prevent vomiting.

**EMG**   *Quick Reference:* Electromyogram. A record of nerve impulses to muscles.
*Advanced Reference:* Involves the responses of the muscles in the diagnosis of nerve conduction defects and muscle contraction.

**Emla**   *Quick Reference:* Topical anaesthetic agent.
*Advanced Reference:* Used for skin analgesia prior to venepuncture, mainly in children but also used with adults. Following application, has an onset of action of approximately 60–90 min. Is a preparation of lignocaine and prilocaine. Particularly useful for patients with needle phobias.

**Emphysema**   *Quick Reference:* (em-fa-seem-a) Abnormal presence of air or gas in the tissues, e.g. lungs and subcutaneous tissue.
*Advanced Reference:* Term normally applied to the lungs in which the alveoli are grossly enlarged and can eventually be destroyed. Found in those suffering from asthma, bronchitis and being associated with smoking and air pollution. The main symptoms are breathlessness. The alveoli can become so damaged that air exchange is barely adequate.

**Empyema**   *Quick Reference:* (em-pie-ema) An internal abscess.
*Advanced Reference:* With empyema the pus occupies a natural cavity within the body, e.g. pleura. Treatment is with drainage and antibiotics.

**Emulsion**   *Quick Reference:* (e-mul-shon) Dispersion of one liquid in another.
*Advanced Reference:* Indicates a preparation in which droplets of one liquid are dispersed in another. Many medicines are prepared in this way.

**Encapsulated**   *Quick Reference:* Contained within a capsule.
*Advanced Reference:* The eye can be described as being within the capsule of the orbital space within the skull. There are other situations where sebaceous cysts form within a fibrous capsule.

**Encapsulectomy**   *Quick Reference:* Removal of the capsule and contents.
*Advanced Reference:* Encapsulectomy is often performed during removal of a sebaceous cyst. The removal of the capsule will minimise the re-occurrence of the cyst.

**Encephalo(n)**   *Quick Reference:* (encef-alo) Relating to the brain.
*Advanced Reference:* Encephalopathy indicates any disease of the brain, especially involving physical changes.

**Endarterectomy**   *Quick Reference:* (en-dar-trec-tommy) Un-blocking of a vessel.

*Advanced Reference:* Commonly refers to an artery (carotid) and the removal of intima and plaque which is causing a blockage. Also referred to as disobliteration.

**Endemic**   *Quick Reference:* Indicates a disease which is always present in the population.

*Advanced Reference:* As opposed to an epidemic which arrives, spreads and disappears.

**Endobronchial**   *Quick Reference:* (endo-bronc-ial) Indicates entering the bronchus.

*Advanced Reference:* Endobronchial tubes and blockers are inserted into the bronchus via the trachea. Both used in thoracic surgery. Blockers are rarely used now whereas endobronchial tubes such as the *Robert-Shaw tube* and Carlens are used regularly for *one-lung anaesthesia*.

**Endocarditis**   *Quick Reference:* Inflammation of the membrane lining the heart (endocardium, the innermost layer of the heart).

*Advanced Reference:* Especially affects the valves of the heart. Acute endocarditis is the result of rheumatic fever. A number of bacteria can also be involved, i.e. *Staphylococcus aureus, S. pneumoniae* or *S. viridans*. Depending on severity, treatment can range from antibiotics to surgical replacement of valves.

**Endocrine**   *Quick Reference:* Term indicating internal secretion.

*Advanced Reference:* An endocrine gland is one which releases its secretion (hormone) directly into the bloodstream to act upon another part of the body.

**Endogenous**   *Quick Reference:* Growing within the body.

*Advanced Reference:* Produced from internal causes, such as disease.

**Endometriosis**   *Quick Reference:* Condition in which endometrium (lining of the uterus) of the uterus is found in abnormal places throughout the body.

*Advanced Reference:* The commonest alternative sites are the surface of the ovaries, peritoneum covering the bladder and pelvic colon, and round ligaments of the uterus. These ectopic fragments pass through the same monthly cycle as the normal uterine membrane, becoming swollen before a period and then bleeding. As there is then no outlet for bleeding this leads to pain during the days prior to a period.

**Endometrium**   *Quick Reference:* (endo-meet-reum) Inner layer of the *uterus*.

*Advanced Reference:* Endometrium is a highly vascular structure that has two distinctive layers. The first layer is the superficial layer within the uterus cavity that sheds itself during menstruation, i.e. stratum *funtionalis*. The deeper layer is permanent offering a vascular supply and reformation of the stratum funtionalis after each menstrual cycle.

**Endorphin**   *Quick Reference:* (en-door-fin) A class of chemical substances found throughout the nervous system.

*Advanced Reference:* Most abundant in the spinal cord and are concerned with sensation and appear to modify the feeling of pain. It is thought that the painkilling action of narcotics may be due to them imitating the natural effect of endorphins, to which they are chemically related. They are produced in response to painful stimuli.

**Endoscope**   *Quick Reference:* Instrument for examining the interior of the body.

*Advanced Reference:* Examples are gastroscope, cystoscope. Can be rigid telescopes or flexible versions which contain fibre-optic light bundles.

**Endoscopy**   *Quick Reference:* Involves the inspection of body cavities, etc. with a telescope.

*Advanced Reference:* A fibre-optic telescope has become the most accepted approach for diagnostic investigations and treatment for looking into the digestive, respiratory, gynaecological, orthopaedic, genito-urinary and neurological systems. The fibre-optic scope is attached to a light source that transmits light through the fibre bundles within the black flexible tubing. In orthopaedic and genito-urinary surgery, the rigid fibre-optic scope is used to give more direct control and manipulation during surgical procedures.

**Endotoxins**   *Quick Reference:* A poison forming part of the bacterium and damaging only tissues in the infected area.

*Advanced Reference:* Found inside bacteria and liberated into the tissues when the organism disintegrates. This is opposed to *exotoxins* which are secreted by the intact bacteria.

**Endotracheal**   *Quick Reference:* Indicates, within the trachea, abbreviated as ET.

*Advanced Reference:* Most commonly refers to the insertion of an ET tube inserted into the trachea during anaesthesia or to provide ventilatory support.

**End plate**   *Quick Reference:* Indicates the motor end plate in the nervous system.

*Advanced Reference:* Located at the terminal membrane of an axon and the post-junctional membrane of the adjoining muscle tissue.

**End tidal**   *Quick Reference:* Applies to gas readings taken at the end of the respiratory cycle.

*Advanced Reference:* End-tidal carbon dioxide ($CO_2$) indicates the reading by the *capnograph* at expiration and is an indication of alveolar $CO_2$ levels.

**End-to-side anastomosis**   *Quick Reference:* Involves anastomosing at one end of a vessel to the side of a larger one.

*Advanced Reference:* Examples would be, jejunum to stomach, donor renal artery to recipient internal iliac artery as in renal transplant.

**Enema**   *Quick Reference:* Substance injected into the rectum.
*Advanced Reference:* Carried out for a variety of reasons, e.g. constipation, washout before operation, to instil nutrients, deliver medication. Also, in radiography when the enema contains barium to outline the rectum and colon.

**Enflurane**   *Quick Reference:* Volatile anaesthetic agent (ethrane).
*Advanced Reference:* Anaesthetic supplement delivered via a calibrated vaporiser. Only a small proportion is metabolised, making it particularly safe for repeated use. Some evidence that it should not be used with *epileptic* patients.

**ENT**   *Quick Reference:* Ear, nose and throat. (otorhinolaryngology).
*Advanced Reference:* Relates to ENT conditions. However, each subject is a speciality in itself.

**Enteral**   *Quick Reference:* The intestine.
*Advanced Reference:* Indicates via the intestinal tract.

**Enterovirus**   *Quick Reference:* A virus which infects the gastrointestinal tract and then the central nervous system.
*Advanced Reference:* They produce specific diseases elsewhere in the body, i.e. polio virus, after entering through the alimentary tract.

**Entonox**   *Quick Reference:* A mixture of *oxygen* and *nitrous oxide* ($N_2O$).
*Advanced Reference:* A mixture of 50% oxygen and 50% $N_2O$. Colour coding is blue and white, cylinders are blue with blue and white quartered shoulders. During storage, cylinders must be laid flat, especially if temperatures are below $-7°C$ in order to avoid the liquid $N_2O$ settling at the bottom of the cylinder, leaving only oxygen above (stratifying). If then used without inverting or shaking the cylinder, only oxygen will be delivered initially followed by pure $N_2O$ once the oxygen is depleted.

**Entropian**   *Quick Reference:* A condition when the eyelid turns inwards.
*Advanced Reference:* More commonly affects the lower eyelid. The eyelashes come into contact with the eye itself. Surgical intervention may include the *excision* of a triangle-shaped piece of skin, muscle and tarsus. The edges are then sutured together to avert the lid margin.

**Enucleation**   *Quick Reference:* To shell out, enucleate.
*Advanced Reference:* Involves the removal of a structure, tumour, gland, etc., as a whole. As with removal of the eye.

**Enzyme**   *Quick Reference:* (en-zime) A substance produced by living cells which promotes chemical change.
*Advanced Reference:* An enzyme is a biological catalyst responsible for metabolism both inside and outside the cells. They are proteins and are specific for one reaction or a well-defined group of similar reactions.

**Epanutin**   *Quick Reference:* Anticonvulsant drug.
*Advanced Reference:* Used to treat grand mal *epileptic* seizures. A preparation of phenytoin.

**Ephedrine**   *Quick Reference:* (ef-e-dreen) Vasoconstrictor and **bronchodilator**.
*Advanced Reference:* Used mainly in the treatment of asthma, chronic bronchitis and *hypotension*, especially during spinal anaesthesia.

**Epicardium**   *Quick Reference:* Outer surface lining of the heart.
*Advanced Reference:* Often referred to as the visceral layer of the serous pericardium. This is a transparent layer with delicate connective tissue that creates a smooth but glossy surface. The glossy surface prevents fibrosis and friction between the adjacent structures within the mediastinum.

**Epidermis**   *Quick Reference:* The outer part of the skin.
*Advanced Reference:* The thin layer of epithelium tissue that is closely connected to the dermis.

**Epididymus**   *Quick Reference:* (epe-did-i-mus) A comma-shaped structure attached to the testis.
*Advanced Reference:* The function of the epididymus is to aid the changes within the spermatozoa. A 6-m length tubing is tightly packed into the comma shape which forms the proximal end of the vas deferens. Research suggests that spermatozoa can be stored within the epididymus potentially for 30 days or longer. After this the spermatozoa is likely to have begun degeneration and become dysfunctional and after this reabsorption begins.

**Epidural**   *Quick Reference:* Indicates a regional anaesthetic technique.
*Advanced Reference:* Refers to the administration of a local anaesthetic (LA) injected outside of the dura, in the thoracic, lumbar or sacral levels of the spinal cord. Used commonly in obstetrics during labour and delivery. Often involves the insertion of an indwelling catheter which is used to top-up the levels of anaesthetic.

**Epigastrium**   *Quick Reference:* A region of the abdomen.
*Advanced Reference:* The upper part of the abdomen in the angle of the ribs over the stomach.

**Epiglottis**   *Quick Reference:* A leaf-shaped cartilage that lies at the back of the tongue.
*Advanced Reference:* The epiglottis covers the opening from the pharynx into the larynx, preventing food from entering the trachea.

**Epilepsy**   *Quick Reference:* The 'falling sickness'
*Advanced Reference:* A convulsive attack due to abnormality of brain function, which may result in a momentary loss of attention or consciousness.

**Episiotomy**   *Quick Reference:* (ep-pes-e-otomy) An incision in the *perineum*.

*Advanced Reference:* The cut is made during childbirth to prevent tearing when the vaginal opening needs to be widened to enable free passage of the baby. Following delivery the cut is sutured.

**Epistaxis**   *Quick Reference:* Bleeding from the nasal cavity.
*Advanced Reference:* May be the result of infection or injury, can be a life-threatening condition if bleeding is excessive and not treated.

**Epontol**   *Quick Reference:* Anaesthetic-induction agent, e.g. propanidid.
*Advanced Reference:* Non-barbiturate anaesthetic-induction agent which has been superseded by newer products. Dissolved in the same solvent (***cremophor***) as *althesin*, therefore had similar reactions and was difficult to inject due to its oily nature. Produces hypotension and hyperventilation followed by apnoea. It is useful for day cases.

**ERCP**   *Quick Reference:* Endoscopic retrograde cholangio pancreatography.
*Advanced Reference:* Involves a combination of endoscopy and contrast radiology may be used to demonstrate the biliary and pancreatic ducts.

**Ergometrine**   *Quick Reference:* Vasoconstrictor and uterine-stimulant drug.
*Advanced Reference:* Used in childbirth during the third stage of labour, for assisting delivery of the placenta and to prevent postnatal bleeding. Commonly used to contract the uterus during termination of pregnancy and Evacuation of Retained Products of Contraception (**ERPC**). Ergot is a fungus which is a parasite of rye and contains numerous alkaloids used in medicine, one being that it directly stimulates involuntary muscle.

**Ergonomics**   *Quick Reference:* The study of efficiency of people in relation to their working environment.
*Advanced Reference:* Vital in lifting and handling in regard to health and safety for both patients and staff.

**Erosion**   *Quick Reference:* The breaking down of tissue usually by ulceration.
*Advanced Reference:* Can refer to a tumour eroding into tissue or a vessel, also erosion of the cervix caused by the replacement of the normal squamous epithelium by columnar epithelium.

**Erythema**   *Quick Reference:* (erith-eem-ea) Reddening of the skin.
*Advanced Reference:* An increased blood flow in the capillaries that may be caused by infection, exposure to cold or an allergic reaction.

**Erythrocyte**   *Quick Reference:* (er-ith-ro-site) A mature red blood cell.
*Advanced Reference:* This red blood cell contains haemoglobin, the substance that transports oxygen from the lungs to the tissues and $CO_2$ from the tissues to the lungs.

**Erythromycin**   *Quick Reference*: (earth-row-mi-sin) antibiotic.

*Advanced Reference:* Used in the treatment of pneumonia, *Legionnaires* disease and as an alternative to penicillin in patients who are *allergic*.

**Escherichea coli**   *Quick Reference:* (es-sher-ekia) An organism commonly found in the intestines.

*Advanced Reference:* Mostly harmless, including *E. coli* which is a normal inhabitant of the large intestine but can cause problems if found in other parts of the body.

**Eschmarch bandage**   *Quick Reference:* (es-mark) A rubber bandage that is rolled onto an arm or leg to produce a bloodless operative field.

*Advanced Reference:* The bandage is applied from the distal end of the limb, with the bandage fully stretched on each turn and overlapping by at least a half inch. Once the bandage reaches the tourniquet cuff, the tourniquet is inflated to the required pressure. Originally functioned as a tourniquet in itself but produces unknown pressures.

**Esmolol**   *Quick Reference:* Anti-arrhythmic.

*Advanced Reference:* Used for the short term treatment of supraventricular arrhythmias (namely, atrial fibrillation, atrial flutter, peri-operative tachycardia).

**ESR**   *Quick Reference:* Erythrocyte sedimentation rate.

*Advanced Reference:* Measures the rate of which red cells settle when a column of blood is left for 1 h.

**Ester**   *Quick Reference:* A class of chemical compounds formed by the bonding of an alcohol and an organic acid.

*Advanced Reference:* A compound formed by mixing alcohol and an acid with the elimination of water. Fats are esters produced by the bonding of fatty acids with the alcohol, glycerol. An esterase is any enzyme that splits esters.

**Ethanol**   *Quick Reference:* Ethyl alcohol.

*Advanced Reference:* Form of alcohol found in alcoholic drinks produced from fermentation of sugar and yeast. Strong solutions are used as an antiseptic and for skin preparation.

**Ethmoid**   *Quick Reference:* (eeth-moid) Sieve like. Small bone of the skull.

*Advanced Reference:* Forms the roof of the nose. Its name refers to the large number of holes for the *olfactory* nerves.

**Ethyl chloride**   *Quick Reference:* (eth-al) Inhalational anaesthetic agent.

*Advanced Reference:* Originally a volatile agent with a rapid onset and highly inflammable. No longer used as an anaesthetic agent but still functional as a (cold) indicator for extent of spread during regional anaesthesia and sometimes used as a topical local anaesthetic, to 'freeze' the area.

**Ethylene oxide**   *Quick Reference:* (eth-leen) A gas used in the sterilisation process.

*Advanced Reference:* Ethylene oxide can penetrate inaccessible parts of a piece of equipment, not able to be sterilised by other methods. However, is explosive and carcinogenic so its use is controlled and also requires a lengthy aeration period.

**Etomidate**   *Quick Reference:* Anaesthetic-induction agent.
*Advanced Reference:* The proprietary form is hypnomidate. A non-barbiturate used mainly because of its lack of cardiovascular-depressant effects.

**Eusol**   *Quick Reference:* (yu-sol) Chlorine-based *antiseptic*.
*Advanced Reference:* Contains hypochlorous and boric acid.

**Eustachian canal**   *Quick Reference:* The connecting tube or channel from the middle ear to the nasopharynx.
*Advanced Reference:* Its purpose is one of equalizing the pressure of the external air and that contained in the middle ear.

**Eustachian tube**   *Quick Reference:* (u-station) A narrow tube that connects the middle ear with the naso-pharynx.
*Advanced Reference:* Its function is to equalise pressure between the middle ear and the atmosphere.

**Evacuator**   *Quick Reference:* A surgical instrument used in urology. Example is Ellicks evacuator.
*Advanced Reference:* Designed to flush out small fragments of stone or tissue shavings from the bladder and prostate.

**Evaporation**   *Quick Reference:* Pertaining to evaporation of a liquid into vapour.
*Advanced Reference:* Applicable especially with reference to heat loss via large incisions during surgery when heat is lost with fluid evaporation. Alcohol-based skin preps also utilise evaporation as the water they are diluted in holds them on the surface until evaporation of the alcohol occurs and this being long enough to lower bacterial count.

**Excretion**   *Quick Reference:* Elimination of by-products of digestion and body chemistry.
*Advanced Reference:* The principal organs of secretion are the kidneys (water, salts, acids, nitrogen compounds), lungs ($CO_2$ and water), skin (water, salt) and liver (bile pigments and salts, poisons).

**Exfoliation**   *Quick Reference:* Peeling of the surface layer.
*Advanced Reference:* Commonly applied to the flaking or peeling of a top surface of skin. Seen routinely in patients who have psoriasis. Can also be used to describe other surface layers such as bone when the cells or enamel surface becomes diseased.

**Exocrine**   *Quick Reference:* A gland with a duct to carry its secretion to its site of action.

*Advanced Reference:* Examples are salivary glands, pancreas to the duodenum. Opposed to *endocrine* which indicates a gland with no duct.

**Exogenous**   *Quick Reference:* Of external origin.

*Advanced Reference:* A condition caused by external factors and environment.

**Exotoxin**   *Quick Reference:* A poisonous substance.

*Advanced Reference:* A soluble poisonous substance produced during growth of a micro-organism and released into the surrounding medium.

**Expiratory valve**   *Quick Reference:* Adjustable pressure-limiting valve.

*Advanced Reference:* A valve, usually within an anaesthetic circuit, which opens to allow passage of expired gas and closes to prevent drawing air in. A common example is the Heidbrink valve which has a thin disc held in place by a spring which in turn is opened or closed by turning a screwed adjuster.

**Extracellular**   *Quick Reference:* Situated or occurring outside of the cells.

*Advanced Reference:* A common reference is extracellular fluid, which indicates all body fluid situated outside of the cells, i.e. intravascualr, interstitial, etc.

**Extradural**   *Quick Reference:* Situated or occurring outside of the *dura* mater but within the skull.

*Advanced Reference:* Epidural indicates placing local anaesthetic outside of the dura and within the epidural space.

**Extrasystoles**   *Quick Reference:* (extra-sist-olee) Indicates extra beats.

*Advanced Reference:* Ectopic beats are an example of extrasystoles.

**Extravasation**   *Quick Reference:* (ex-trav-a-sachun) Escape of fluid from a (blood) vessel into the tissues.

*Advanced Reference:* Occurs when a needle or cannula 'tissues' or 'extravasates'. Should the drug or medicine being injected have the potential for harm, there are agents which can help to disperse and/or increase absorption, e.g. *hyaluronidase.*

**Extremity**   *Quick Reference:* Indicates the distal part.

*Advanced Reference:* Refers to the hand or foot and more usually, the fingers and toes.

**Extubation**   *Quick Reference:* The removal of an ET tube.

*Advanced Reference:* General term used for the removal of all types and designs of tube from the trachea, etc., either in the theatre, recovery or intensive therapy unit (ITU) setting.

**Exudate**   *Quick Reference:* A discharge of serous fluid.

*Advanced Reference:* It is composed of fluid, cells and debris which due to inflammation has escaped from the blood vessels into the tissues.

**Face mask (anaesthetic)**   *Quick Reference:* The face mask connects the patient to the breathing system and anaesthetic machine.

*Advanced Reference:* The anaesthetic face mask is made of black rubber and/or transparent plastic, with an inflatable cuff to ensure a snug fit over the face. It is designed to contour itself to the face and is available in several different sizes. The proximal end of the mask has a 22-mm inlet for connection to the angle piece. The angle piece fits to a catheter mount and/or a breathing system.

Designs include 'Ambu' and 'Rendell-Baker'. The 'goldman' mask is a nasal inhaler which is often used in dental chair anaesthesia.

Excessive pressure by the mask may cause injury to structures of the face, e.g. the branches of the *trigeminal* or facial nerves. It can also cause an increase in 'dead space' of up to 200 ml in adults.

Other masks used in anaesthetics/recovery include the *variable performance masks* (medium concentration (MC) mask) which give oxygen-enriched air to the patient and the *Venturi* masks which are fixed performance and give specific oxygen concentration to the patient.

**Faciomaxillary**   *Quick Reference:* Refers to the surgical speciality dealing with facial injury and deformity.

*Advanced Reference:* Also referred to as maxillo-facial, or in slang terms 'max-fax'. Involves features of dentistry/orthodontics, ear, nose and throat (ENT), orthopaedic and plastic surgery.

**Fahrenheit**   *Quick Reference:* (far-en-height) Temperature-measuring scale.

*Advanced Reference:* Sets the freezing point of water at 32° and boiling point at 212°. Body temperature using this scale is 98.4°.

**Failed intubation**   *Quick Reference:* Indicates a patient not being able to be intubated following a number of attempts.

*Advanced Reference:* Often confused with difficult intubation but whereas this involves the reasons that may cause intubation to be difficult, failed intubation usually involves a policy or guidelines of what should be done in this situation. Commonly involves aspects such as how many attempts should be made before considering alternatives, as well as the assistant maintaining cricoid pressure, etc.

**Falciform**   *Quick Reference:* (fals-e-form) Sickle-shaped ligament within the hepatic system.

*Advanced Reference:* A fold of peritoneum connected to the anterior abdominal wall and diaphragm and which separates the two lobes of the liver.

**Fallopian tubes**   *Quick Reference:* Bilateral tubes which run from the ovaries to the upper corners of the uterus.

*Advanced Reference:* They are lined with ciliated epithelium which collects the egg from the ovaries and propels it down the tube into the uterus. If fertilisation takes place but the ovum does not travel to the uterus, an ectopic pregnancy can occur in the fallopian tube.

**Fallot's tetralogy**   *Quick Reference:* **Congenital** heart condition.

*Advanced Reference:* This condition has four component defects; an opening in the interventricular *septum*, the partition between the right and left ventricles, a narrowing of the valve of the *pulmonary* artery, over-development of the right ventricle and displacement of the aorta to the right. A child suffering from this condition is *cyanosed* due to the circulating blood not being properly oxygenated.

**Faradic stimulation**   *Quick Reference:* Electric current applied to a muscle. Faradism.

*Advanced Reference:* Physiotherapy technique where muscles are made to contract by the application of an intermittent current when patients are unable to contract the muscle voluntarily. Used sometimes in obstetrics and gynaecology to stimulate the muscles of the pelvis which have become lax usually following childbirth.

**Fascia**   *Quick Reference:* (fash-ia) Fibrous tissue wrapped around muscles and organs.

*Advanced Reference:* Referred to as the packing material of the body. Found throughout the body, e.g. as the periosteum covering bones which merges with fascial sheaths of neighbouring muscles. Lies just under the skin as the superficial and deep fascia. The superficial contains fat, nerves and blood vessels while the deep is densely fibrous.

**Fasciectomy**   *Quick Reference:* (fash-e-ectomy) Removal of fascia.

*Advanced Reference:*The most common procedure is palmer fasciectomy due to contracture (***Dupuytren's***) of fingers.

**Fasiculation**   *Quick Reference:* (fas-ic-you-lay-hun) Flickering or twitching of muscle.

*Advanced Reference:* Reaction produced when muscle relaxant suxamethonium is injected. Fasiculation occurs as the drug produces ***depolarisation.***

**FASIER**   *Quick Reference:* Follicle aspiration sperm injection and assisted rupture. Type of infertility treatment.

*Advanced Reference:* Carried out under ultrasound guidance and used to remove the egg directly from a follicle. Next the sperm and egg are mixed inside the syringe and then injected into the patient.

**Fat embolism**   *Quick Reference:* Fatty deposit entering the blood circulation.
*Advanced Reference:* Most common after orthopaedic procedures such as hip replacement when reaming of the bone has been carried out.

**Fatty liver disease**   *Quick Reference:* Also called steatosis. It is a build-up of fat in liver cells.
*Advanced Reference:* Caused by long-term alcohol abuse. Along with hepatitis and cirrhosis, it is one of the three primary types of alcohol-induced liver disease.

**Fazadinium**   *Quick Reference:* Non-depolarising neuromuscular-blocking drug.
*Advanced Reference:* Onset of action is approximately 1 min and this is why it was thought to be an alternative to suxamethonium.

**Febrile**   *Quick Reference:* Related to fever.
*Advanced Reference:* Associated with *pyrexia.* Febrile convulsions in children are caused by fever.

**Feeding tube**   *Quick Reference:* Refers to invasive catheters, etc. inserted into the body to provide nutrition.
*Advanced Reference:* The term commonly applies to total parenteral nutrition (*TPN*) lines (Nutri-Cath), etc. inserted into a central vein rather than direct *gastrostomy* tubes, etc. Inserted when the patient cannot take nutrition normally (enteric route) due to obstruction, removal of sections of the gastrointestinal tract or when on long-term ventilation in intensive therapy unit (*ITU*).

**Femoro-popliteal bypass**   *Quick Reference:* Vascular surgery procedure.
*Advanced Reference:* Involves the restoration of blood flow to the leg with a graft bypassing the occluded section of the femoral artery.

**Femur**   *Quick Reference:* The thigh bone.
*Advanced Reference:* Said to be the largest and strongest bone in the human body. At the upper end its rounded head fits into the acetabulum (cup-shaped socket) of the *pelvis* to form a ball and socket joint while its lower end forms a joint at the knee.

**Fenestra**   *Quick Reference:* A window or opening.
*Advanced Reference:* A common example is the opening between the middle and inner ear.

**Fenestrated tracheostomy tube**   *Quick Reference:* Curved plastic tube used to assist in breathing, the fenestration allows the patient to speak.

*Advanced Reference: **Tracheostomy*** tubes are used for intermittent positive pressure ventilation (IPPV), upper airway obstruction, maintenance of an airway and long-term control of bronchial secretions.

A tracheostomy tube is composed of an introducer, wings for attachment of securing tape, inflatable cuff (usually), 15 mm connector (usually) on proximal end.

Complications of use can include ***haemorrhage***, occlusion, infection and ulceration of the trachea.

The fenestrated tube allows the patient to speak by channelling air to the *vocal cords*.

**Fenestration**   *Quick Reference:* Making an opening or window.

*Advanced Reference*: An ENT procedure designed to assist hearing when deafness is due to otosclerosis. Involves making an opening in the bony labyrinth of the ear.

**Fentanyl**   *Quick Reference:* (fent-an-il) A narcotic analgesic, e.g. ***sublimaze***.

*Advanced Reference:* Synthetic analgesic derived from *pethidine*. Used as a supplement during anaesthesia. It is a powerful respiratory depressant.

**Fentazin**   *Quick Reference:* Perphenazine. Primarily an antipsychotic drug.

*Advanced Reference:* Used to treat anxiety or as an anti-emetic prior to surgery.

**Ferric**   *Quick Reference:* Ferrous or iron.

*Advanced Reference:* Ferrous sulphate is used to treat iron-deficiency anaemia. Other preparations include ferrous succinate and fumarate.

**FESS**   *Quick Reference:* Functional endoscopic sinus surgery. ***Endoscopic*** examination of the sinus cavity within the skull.

*Advanced Reference:* The insertion of a fine telescope into the nasal or other skull cavity to determine the cause of blocked sinuses.

**Fibre-optics**   *Quick Reference:* Refers to the light-carrying system used in fibrescopes.

*Advanced Reference:* Utilises glass or plastic fibres to carry images and light, which also means that the instrument has a degree of flexibility and so more readily introduced into the body than rigid scopes.

**Fibrillation**   *Quick Reference:* Rapid uncoordinated contractions of the heart muscle.

*Advanced Reference:* May be atrial (AF) or ventricular (VF). Produces an ineffective pumping action of the heart.

**Fibrinogen**   *Quick Reference:* An ***enzyme*** involved in the clotting of blood.

*Advanced Reference:* Fibrinogen is a soluble protein dissolved in the plasma and is converted into threads of an insoluble protein, fibrin, which forms a mesh and eventually becomes a clot after serum has been squeezed out.

**Fibrin sealant**   *Quick Reference:* Biological tissue glue composed of *thrombin* and *fibrinogen* used to stop air leaks and control bleeding.

   *Advanced Reference:* Applied topically to help stop bleeding. The main active ingredient is fibrinogen and works by forming a flexible covering over the oozing blood vessel and can control bleeding within 5 min.

**Fibroadenoma**   *Quick Reference:* Solid benign lump in the breast.

   *Advanced Reference:* Mostly painless and mobile. However, may cause discomfort and become larger, especially during pregnancy. Can be removed surgically if necessary.

**Fibroid**   *Quick Reference:* (fibe-roid) Overgrowth of muscle and connective tissue in the wall of the uterus.

   *Advanced Reference:* Described as smooth muscle tumours, usually benign and can vary in size. Can cause pain, pressure on adjacent organs, vaginal bleeding and infertility. May be treated conservatively or with surgery.

**Fibrosarcoma**   *Quick Reference:* Type of soft tissue sarcoma.

   *Advanced Reference:* A malignant tumour of fibrous tissue which grows relatively slowly often in muscles near the surface of the body. Can invade neighbouring tissue and metastasise the lungs.

**Fibrosis**   *Quick Reference:* Growth of scar tissue.

   *Advanced Reference:* Can be due to infection, inflammatory injury, or even healing. Common conditions include cystic fibrosis and pulmonary fibrosis.

**Fibrositis**   *Quick Reference:* Inflammation of fibrous tissue.

   *Advanced Reference:* Involves pain and stiffness. Common sites affected are the back and neck. Sometimes referred to as muscular rheumatism.

**Filters**   *Quick Reference:* Devices used to remove substances from gases and fluids.

   *Advanced Reference:* Filters are used within breathing systems to remove bacteria and prevent cross infection. Positioned usually as close to the patient end as possible in an anaesthetic circuit and at the inlet tubing to ventilators. Blood filters are designed to remove micro-aggregates during transfusion. These have formed during the storage period from *platelets*, *leucocytes* and *fibrins* and are suspected to be a cause of pulmonary micro-*embolism.* Further examples of filters are *drawing-up needles* that contain filters intended to prevent minute particles from glass vials being injected and *in-line bacterial epidural filters.*

**Finger cot**   *Quick Reference:* A small finger glove.

   *Advanced Reference:* Finger cots were used to perform rectal examinations.

**Fissure**   *Quick Reference:* (fish-ure) A cleft or groove in a structure.

   *Advanced Reference:* A common example is an anal fissure, which is a crack in the mucous membrane of the anus often caused by hard faeces.

**Fistula**   *Quick Reference:* A pipe or tube. Plural is fistulae.

*Advanced Reference:* An abnormal connection between the cavity of one organ with another or the surface of the body. Examples include vesico-vaginal (urinary bladder and vagina), fistula in ano (anal canal and skin) and an atrioventricular (AV) fistula (artery and vein).

**Fitzpatrick**   *Quick Reference:* System for classifying skin types by their colour and response to sunlight.

*Advanced Reference:* Involves the amount of melanin a person has in their epidermis. The classification covers 1–6 types from those who always sunburn to dark/black skin types who cannot burn.

**Fixation**   *Quick Reference:* To render something stable or immovable.

*Advanced Reference:* Usually applied to the repair and stabilisation of bones and joints.

**Flagyl**   *Quick Reference:* (flag-il) Antibacterial preparation.

*Advanced Reference:* Proprietary form of the amoebicidal drug metronidazole with high activity against anaerobic bacteria. Available as an infusion for intravenous (IV) use.

**Flail chest**   *Quick Reference:* Chest injury involving broken ribs or sternum.

*Advanced Reference:* The fracture causes disruption to the normal functioning of the thorax in that the broken section becomes detached and no longer moves outwards on inspiration but is drawn inwards by negative pressure and is pushed outwards during expiration while the rest of the thorax contracts.

**Flamazine**   *Quick Reference:* Proprietary antibacterial cream.

*Advanced Reference:* Used to treat wounds, burns, ulcers, bedsores and skin graft donor sites. It is a preparation of silver sulphadiazine in a water-soluble base.

**Flap**   *Quick Reference:* Usually refers to a section of tissue used for grafting.

*Advanced Reference:* The flap is left attached to its blood supply and can be used to repair defects either close by or some distance from the donor site.

**Flexion**   *Quick Reference:* Indicates bending.

*Advanced Reference:* The movement of bending a joint. Opposite to extension. A flexor muscle is any muscle that causes the bending of a limb or other body part.

**Floating ribs**   *Quick Reference:* Refers to the last pairs of ribs.

*Advanced Reference:* These are connected only to the vertebrae but not the sternum as are the rest of the ribs.

**Flowmeter**   *Quick Reference:* A flowmeter measures the flow of gas through them and are always used on anaesthetic machines.

*Advanced Reference:* Flowmeters measure the flow rate of a gas passing through them. They are individually calibrated at room temperature and atmospheric pressure for each gas. In the anaesthetic machine, the flow rate is measured in litres per minute.

The flowmeter consists of a flow control valve, a tapered plastic tube (wider at the top) and a lightweight bobbin.

When the needle valve is opened, gas enters the tapered tube. The bobbin is kept floating within the tube by the gas flow passing around it. The higher the flow rate, the higher the bobbin rises. A rotating bobbin indicates that it is floating and not just stuck in position.

Dangers in use include flowmeters sticking (caused by, e.g. dirt or static electricity) and giving the wrong reading, pressure rise at the common gas outlet can result in wrong readings.

**Floxapen**   *Quick Reference:* Proprietary antibiotic.
*Advanced Reference:* Used in the treatment of skin and ENT infections, especially those caused by *Staphylcoccus* and have become resistant to penicillin, e.g. flucloxacillin.

**Fluid balance**   *Quick Reference:* Relates to the intake and output of fluids usually on a daily basis.
*Advanced Reference:* Average adult daily intake is approximately 1500 mls daily but can vary with climate etc. Output involves the fluid in urine, faeces, sweat, evaporation,etc. Surgical patients fluid balance must be monitored effectively by including loss from fasting, bleeding, urinary output, evaporation etc. Input during surgery is mainly through intravenous methods.

**Fluid retention**   *Quick Reference:* Failure to excrete excess fluid from the body.
*Advanced Reference:* May be due to renal, cardiovascular or metabolic disorders.

**Flumazenil**   *Quick Reference:* Benzodiazepine antagonist.
*Advanced Reference:* Also known as anexate. Reverses the sedative effects of the benzodiazepine group of drugs.

**Fluoroscope**   *Quick reference:* Viewing screen used in radiology/radiography.
*Advanced Reference:* It is a fluorescent screen which enables images to be viewed directly rather than taking X-ray films.

**Flutter**   *Quick Reference:* Refers to an irregular heartbeat, an arrhythmia.
*Advanced Reference:* Atrial flutter, referred to as 'saw-tooth' when viewed on an electrocardiographical (*ECG*) trace. Due to rapid atrial discharge and can be up to 300 per minute. In relation to theatre can be caused by insertion of a central venous pressure (*CVP*) line, *hypovolaemia*, *pulmonary embolism*. Treated with *cardioversion*, pacing and drug therapy (*digoxin*, *amiodarone*, *verapamil*).

**Foetus**   *Quick Reference:* (fe-tus) Unborn offspring developing in the uterus.
*Advanced Reference:* Also has a spelling of fetus. Before the 8th week and after conception the child is called an embryo but between the 8th week and the end of pregnancy is referred to as the foetus.

**Follicle**   *Quick Reference:* A very small secreting gland.
*Advanced Reference:* In the ovary the ovum develops in a small cystic space filled with fluid called a graffian follicle. Follicle-stimulating hormone (FSH) is one of the hormones of the anterior *pituitary* gland, which stimulates the formation of the ovum in the ovary and spermatozoa in the testis.

**Fontanelle**   *Quick Reference:* (font-an-el) Space between the cranial bones of an infant.
*Advanced Reference:* When first born, a baby's skull bones have not completely come together and there are six places where the gaps are closed by membrane. The largest is on top of the head where the frontal bone and the two parietal bones at the sides leave a gap of approximately a square inch and this is called the anterior fontanelle. This gap usually closes by about 18 months.

**Foramen**   *Quick Reference:* An opening or hole.
*Advanced Reference:* A natural opening especially into or through bone for the passage of blood vessels or nerves. The largest is the foramen magnum at the base of the skull through which the spinal cord passes into the vertebral column.

**Foreign body**   *Quick Reference:* Anything found within the body which is not naturally there.
*Advanced Reference:* Can be within the digestive tract, lungs, etc., either swallowed or inhaled. Many need to be removed surgically.

**Foreskin**   *Quick Reference:* (for-skin) Skin covering the end of the penis.
*Advanced Reference:* The prepuce. Covers the glans penis and its inner surface secretes a lubricating fluid.

**Formaldehyde**   *Quick Reference:* (for-mal-dee-hide) A pungent gas soluble in water.
*Advanced Reference:* Used as a powerful disinfectant and for sterilising instruments that cannot withstand heat. Available in tablet form which gives off a strong and irritant vapour. Also used in a water solution as formalin as a fixative for laboratory specimens.

**Forrester spray**   *Quick Reference:* Throat spray.
*Advanced Reference:* Design of throat spray used in anaesthetics to deliver local anaesthetic (LA).

**Fortral**   *Quick Reference:* Proprietary narcotic analgesic.
*Advanced Reference:* The active constituent is the opiate pentazocine.

**Fossa**   *Quick Reference:* A depression or hollow area.

*Advanced Reference:* Many are found in or are related to bones such as the *iliac fossa* which is the depression on the inner surface of the iliac bone. The *cubital fossa* is the triangular depression at the front of the elbow where veins are sometimes used for IV cannulation.

**Fothergill's operation**   *Quick Reference:* Gynaecological operation.

*Advanced Reference:* An operation carried out to correct prolapse of the uterus. Involves amputation of the cervix with anterior and posterior *colporrhaphy*.

**Frenulum**   *Quick Reference:* Section of tissue which limits the movement of an organ.

*Advanced Reference:* Is a fold of mucous membrane as in the fold under the tongue or that at the back of the penis.

**Fresh-frozen plasma**   *Quick Reference:* FFP.

*Advanced Reference:* Frozen plasma is rich in *factor VIII* and *fibrinogen*, used commonly during multiple transfusion.

**Friable**   *Quick Reference:* Indicates that a substance (tissue) crumbles easy.

*Advanced Reference:* Term used in relation to tissues which due to their texture are difficult to repair or diathermize, as with the liver and so bleeding is difficult to control.

**Frozen section**   *Quick Reference:* Tissue biopsy taken during surgery for examination.

*Advanced Reference:* When a frozen section is to be taken, pre-arrangements are made with the laboratory and a pathology form is completed in advance by the surgeon. Immediately the biopsy is taken, it is placed in a dry pot and transported immediately to the laboratory. Results take approximately 20–30 min and are phoned through directly to the theatre and surgeon.

**Fulguration**   *Quick Reference:* Cautery.

*Advanced Reference:* The application of diathermy to destroy unwanted areas of tissues, warts, growths, skin tags, etc.

**Full blood count**   *Quick Reference:* FBC. Blood screening carried out to ascertain (normal) state of a patient's blood.

*Advanced Reference:* Involves blood grouping, cross-matching (X-matching), clotting times, haemoglobin (Hb) levels, urea and electrolytes (U&E), etc.

**Fulminating**   *Quick Reference:* Sudden.

*Advanced Reference:* In reference to a disease or condition, indicates sudden onset and rapid progress.

**Fumigation**   *Quick Reference:* Process of burning or volatilising substances.
*Advanced Reference:* Carried out to produce vapours which destroy infective organisms and vermin.

**Fundoplication**   *Quick reference:* Surgical procedure. Nissen fundoplication is the wrapping of the fundus of the stomach around the oesophagus at the gastric–oesophageal junction.
*Advanced Reference:* Indicated for severe gastro-oesophageal reflux. Commonly in children who have an inadequate anti-reflux barrier.

**Fundus**   *Quick Reference:* The part of a hollow remote from its opening.
*Advanced Reference:* The base of an organ. The top of the uterus furthest from the cervix.

**Fungus**   *Quick Reference:* A simple kind of plant life.
*Advanced Reference:* Closely related to bacteria. Are parasites that live on other plants and animals. The cause of fungal diseases, usually superficial infections of the skin (ringworm) and mucous membrane (thrush). Moulds and yeasts are examples. Some antibiotics are produced by moulds.

**Fusion**   *Quick Reference:* Surgical *fixation* of a joint.
*Advanced Reference:* An example is spinal fusion which involves bridging adjacent vertebrae with a bone graft to prevent movement.

# G

**Gallamine** *Quick Reference:* (galla-mean) Non-depolarising muscle relaxant, e.g. flaxedil.

*Advanced Reference:* Rarely used now, causes tachycardia, not used in obstetrics as it readily crosses the *placenta* and not suitable for renal failure patients as it is almost entirely excreted by the kidneys.

**Gall bladder** *Quick Reference:* Small bag attached to the underside of the liver.

*Advanced Reference:* Pear shaped with muscular walls, stores and concentrates bile (gall) then discharges it to the *duodenum* via the cystic duct.

**Gallipot** *Quick Reference:* A small pot for holding lotions, etc. during surgery.

*Advanced Reference:* Often used in conjunction with kidney dishes (receivers). Used to hold prepping solutions or sutures and small items that could become misplaced during surgery.

**Gallstones:** *Quick Reference:* Stones found in the *gall bladder.*

*Advanced Reference:* Found generally in the biliary tract. There are three types: cholesterol stones, bile pigment stones and mixed stones of all plus calcium.

**Galvonometer** *Quick Reference:* Instrument for detecting and measuring small electric currents.

*Advanced Reference:* Works on the principle of an interaction between an electric current and a magnetic field.

**Gamma globulin** *Quick Reference:* Type of blood protein.

*Advanced Reference:* They are antibodies responsible for immunity to specific infections.

**Gamma rays** *Quick Reference:* Ionising radiation. Electromagnetic rays.

*Advanced Reference:* This form of ionising radiation has rays of shorter wavelength and greater penetration than X-rays. Used in both radiotherapy and sterilisation of medical products and devices.

**Ganglion**   *Quick Reference:* Collection of nerve cells or cystic swelling.
*Advanced Reference:* Refers to a network of nerves outside of the central nervous system (*CNS*). Alternatively, a painless cyst-like swelling found in tendon sheath or joint capsule, often at the wrist.

**Gangrene**   *Quick Reference:* (gan-green) Death of tissue.
*Advanced Reference:* Usually due to inadequate blood supply because of arterial disease or injury which is commonly referred to as dry gangrene, whereas wet gangrene is more often due to bacterial infection.

**Garamycin**   *Quick Reference:* (gara-my-sin) Type of *antibiotic*.
*Advanced Reference:* Used primarily in the form of drops to treat bacterial infections of the ear and eye.

**Gas laws**   *Quick Reference:* Refers to those laws and principles related to patient physiology and functioning of related equipment.
*Advanced Reference:* Mainly the following: (i) *Boyle's law* states that at a constant temperature, the volume of mass of gas is inversely proportional to the pressure. (ii) *Dalton's law* states that the pressure exerted by a fixed amount of a gas in a mixture equals the pressure it would exert if alone; thus the pressure exerted by a mixture of gases equals the sum of the partial pressures exerted by each gas. (iii) *Charle's law* states that the coefficient of expansion of any gas at a constant pressure is 1/273. (iv) *Henry's law* states that the amount of gas dissolved in a solvent is proportional to its partial pressure above the solvent, at constant temperature.

**Gastrectomy**   *Quick Reference:* Partial or total removal of the stomach.
*Advanced Reference:* Partial gastrectomy involves excision of various parts and portions depending on site and type of lesion or spread of disease. The common procedures are Billroth types 1 and 2 and Polya.

**Gastric**   *Quick Reference:* Pertaining to the stomach.
*Advanced Reference:* Used in relation to the stomach, i.e. gastric juice, gastric ulcer, etc.

**Gastrin**   *Quick Reference:* Hormone released into the blood by the stomach.
*Advanced Reference:* Released by the lower end of the stomach in response to the presence of protein foods and stimulates acid release from the upper stomach.

**Gastro-enteritis**   *Quick Reference:* Inflammation of the stomach and intestine.
*Advanced Reference:* Commonly due to bacterial or viral infection (food poisoning). Characterised by vomiting, pain and diarrhoea.

**Gastro-enterostomy**   *Quick Reference:* Surgical opening between the stomach and small intestine.

*Advanced Reference:* Usually performed because of obstruction of the *pylorus*.

**Gastrojejunostomy**   *Quick Reference:* Opening made between the stomach and upper loop of *jejunum.*

*Advanced Reference:* Performed usually for pyloric obstruction so that food can pass directly from the stomach into the upper part of the small intestine. Gastroduodenostomy is the surgical creation of an anastomosis between the stomach and the duodenum.

**Gastroscope**   *Quick Reference:* Illuminated tube passed down the esophagus for examination.

*Advanced Reference:* A flexible instrument as opposed to a rigid oesophagoscope.

**Gastrostomy**   *Quick Reference:* Opening between the stomach and the overlying abdominal wall.

*Advanced Reference:* Used when the oesophagus is blocked or the patient is unable to swallow. A self-retaining feeding tube is introduced into the opening.

**Gelatin**   *Quick Reference:* Colourless, transparent substance made from animal collagen.

*Advanced Reference:* Used mostly in medicine for drug capsules or suppositories.

**Gelofucin**   *Quick Reference:* (jelo-fusin) Intravenous (IV) plasma expander.

*Advanced Reference:* Form of gelatin from animal protein. Used as an infusion to expand the overall blood volume. Can produce allergic reactions.

**Gene**   *Quick Reference:* (jean) A factor which controls the inheritance of a specific characteristic.

*Advanced Reference:* One of the hereditary factors in the chromosome and helps to determine physical and mental makeup.

**Generic**   *Quick Reference:* The official name of a drug.

*Advanced Reference:* This is opposed to the brand or proprietary name given by a particular manufacturer.

**Genital**   *Quick Reference:* Refers to the organs of reproduction.

*Advanced Reference:* Genitalia.

**Gentamicin**   *Quick Reference:* A broad-spectrum antibiotic.

*Advanced Reference:* Used to treat many forms of infection, namely urinary tract, meningitis, endocarditis, septicaemia. Administered by injection or topical route as not capable of being absorbed by the digestive system via oral tablet.

**Gentian violet**   *Quick Reference:* (gen-shan) An antiseptic dye.
*Advanced Reference:* Used to treat bacterial and fungal skin infections, abrasions, etc. Also available as a skin prep in surgery and used to stain specimens for microscopical examination.

**Geriatrics**   *Quick Reference:* Branch of medicine that deals with disease of the aged.
*Advanced Reference:* Also studies the problems of growing old, and causes and nature of related diseases and conditions.

**Gestation**   *Quick Reference:* Period between conception and birth.
*Advanced Reference:* Gestation in women is calculated from the beginning of the last menstrual period and has a duration of approximately 40 weeks.

**Gingiva**   *Quick Reference:* The soft tissue of the gums.
*Advanced Reference:* Gingivitis is inflammation of the gums due to bacterial infection.

**Girdlestone**   *Quick Reference:* Operation performed for osteo-arthritis.
*Advanced Reference:* Involves excision of the head of the femur and part of the *acetabulum* followed by the suturing of a mass of muscle between the bone ends.

**Girth**   *Quick Reference:* Circumference.
*Advanced Reference:* May be pertaining to the abdomen when girth measurements are important following trauma. Increasing measurement could indicate internal haemorrhage.

**Giving-set**   *Quick Reference:* Standard term for a blood-transfusion set.
*Advanced Reference:* Also termed 'drip set', which is a general term whereas 'giving-set' refers to the particular design for blood transfusion as opposed to fluid administration sets.

**Gland**   *Quick Reference:* An organ that forms and releases substances that act elsewhere in the body.
*Advanced Reference:* If the secretion is carried to the surface of the body or lining of a hollow organ it is termed exocrine (digestive glands and sweat glands). If it is carried in the bloodstream it is termed endocrine (pituitary and thyroid).

**Glasgow coma scale**   *Quick Reference:* Scale developed to assess head-injured patients.
*Advanced reference:* Although devised for head-injured patients, the scale is also applied to the recovery ward for assessing general conscious state. It is also used to record the depth of coma, i.e. the lower the score, the more deeply unconscious the patient.

**Glaucoma**   *Quick Reference:* (glore-coma) A disease of the eye.
*Advanced Reference:* Occurs usually after middle age. The pressure of the fluid inside the eye rises and damages the optic nerve and the retina because drainage of aqueous humour is blocked.

**Glomerulonephritis**   *Quick Reference:* Inflammation of the glomeruli of the kidney.
*Advanced Reference:* Formerly known as Bright's disease. An acute condition usually following streptococcal infection.

**Glomerulus**   *Quick Reference:* Tangle of minute blood vessels in the kidney.
*Advanced Reference:* The glomerulus is sited inside the **Bowman's capsule** and is involved in the filtration of the blood in the process of urine formation.

**Glossitis**   *Quick Reference:* Glosso is a prefix indicating the tongue.
*Advanced Reference:* Glossitis is inflammation of the surface of the tongue.

**Glossopharyngeal nerve**   *Quick Reference:* The ninth cranial nerve.
*Advanced Reference:* Contains both motor and sensory fibres supplying muscles of the throat, **parotid** *salivary glands* and relays sensation from the throat, tonsil and back part of the tongue, including the sense of taste. Also, carries sensation from the middle ear and **carotid** body.

**Glottis**   *Quick Reference:* Part of the **larynx**.
*Advanced Reference:* The area which contains the vocal cords where the voice is produced.

**Glove powder**   *Quick Reference:* Talc-like substance included with surgical gloves to aid donning and removal.
*Advanced Reference:* Suspected of causing tissue inflammation and being responsible for post-operative adhesions. Also, the method of applying the powder allowed it to become airborne and so lead to respiratory tract irritation in staff.

**Glucagon**   *Quick Reference:* Hormone secreted by the pancreas.
*Advanced Reference:* This hormone instigates a rise in circulating blood sugar by increasing the release of glucose from the liver.

**Glucose**   *Quick Reference:* A simple sugar.
*Advanced Reference:* Combustion of glucose and oxygen forms water and carbon dioxide which is the principal source of energy in the body.

**Glucose reagent sticks**   *Quick Reference:* Product used to measure glucose concentration.
*Advanced Reference:* Usually made of plastic with a reagent tip and used to measure blood or urine glucose concentration. Useful more as a guide than accurate measurement. Sometimes referred to product names of Dextro-sticks, Lab-sticks or Multi-Sticks.

**Glue**   *Quick Reference:* Surgical glue for wound healing.
　　*Advanced Reference:* A bioadhesive glue used for superficial wounds.

**Glue ear**   *Quick Reference:* Otitis media.
　　*Advanced Reference:* Occurs in children and can lead to deafness as the middle ear becomes blocked by sticky thick material which interferes with the movement of the *ossicles.* Treatment involves placement of a *grommet* into the ear drum to allow ventilation of the middle ear.

**Gluteal**   *Quick Reference:* Pertaining to an area of the buttocks.
　　*Advanced Reference:* The fleshy area of the buttocks is formed by three muscles.

**Gluten**   *Quick Reference:* A protein found in cereals.
　　*Advanced Reference:* People with *coeliac* disease cannot tolerate gluten and should eat a gluten-free diet.

**Gluteraldehyde**   *Quick Reference:* A disinfectant and chemical sterilising agent.
　　*Advanced Reference:* Closely related to formaldehyde. Referred to commonly by its brand name, Cidex and used in the sterilisation of instruments. Has been replaced with safer products as Health and Safety Regulations highlighted the hazards of inhalation and contact.

**Glycerol**   *Quick Reference:* (glis-erol) Mixture of fat and oils. Also termed glycerin.
　　*Advanced Reference:* Used in many skin preparations, as a sweetening agent in medicines and as a laxative in anal suppositories.

**Glyceryl trinitrate**   *Quick Reference:* Vasodilator drug also known as nitroglycerine (GTN).
　　*Advanced Reference:* Used in the relief of angina, relaxes smooth muscle and dilates the blood vessels. Available as sublingual tablets and skin patches. Also available in ampoules (tridil) and infused during surgery to lower blood pressure.

**Glycine**   *Quick Reference:* Irrigating solution used in urological procedures.
　　*Advanced Reference:* Used as a 1.5% solution during trans-urethral resection of the prostate, tumour and bladder neck resection (*TURP*, TURT, TURBN, respectively), etc.

**Glycogen**   *Quick Reference:* A carbohydrate, starch.
　　*Advanced Reference:* Formed from *glucose* and stored in the liver and muscles as an energy reserve to be called on as needed. As glucose is used up, glycogen is converted at the same rate so that glucose levels remain constant.

**Goitre**   *Quick Reference:* (goy-ta) Enlargement of the *thyroid* gland.

*Advanced Reference:* Simple goitres are attributed to iodine deficiency and do not involve over- or under-activity of the thyroid itself. Treatment is by surgical removal.

**Golden hour**   *Quick Reference:* Term related to emergency aid/medicine.
*Advanced Reference:* Refers to the first hour of injury when immediate advanced care is known to extend survival rates. Introduced initially with heart attack patients.

**Goldman**   *Quick Reference:* Name associated with a number of anaesthetic devices.
*Advanced Reference:* Most commonly there is the Goldman draw-over vaporiser and Goldman nasal mask/inhaler used primarily in dental anaesthesia.

**Gonadotropia**   *Quick Reference:* **Hormone** formed in the *pituitary gland.*
*Advanced Reference:* Hormone that acts on the **gonads.** Also as chorionic gonadotropin suppresses the mothers' menstrual cycle during pregnancy.

**Gonads**   *Quick Reference:* Primary sex organs.
*Advanced Reference:* Indicates the ovary or testis.

**Gonorrhoea**   *Quick Reference:* (gone-or-ea) A sexually transmitted venereal disease.
*Advanced Reference:* Caused by the *Gonococcus* bacteria which invades the mucous membranes of the urethra and can also invade the uterus. Can often be the cause of male urethral strictures.

**Gordon-Greene tube**   *Quick Reference:* Endobronchial tube.
*Advanced Reference:* The Gordon-Green tube has a slot for the right upper lobe bronchus and a carinal hook.

**Gouge**   *Quick Reference:* Orthopaedic surgical instrument.
*Advanced Reference:* A type of chisel of curved design used for scooping out bone.

**Gout**   *Quick Reference:* High level of uric acid in the blood.
*Advanced Reference:* Causes painful inflammation of a joint, the big toe joints being commonly affected.

**Graefe's knife**   *Quick Reference:* Fine pointed knife used in ophthalmology.
*Advanced Reference:* Used to make an incision into the **limbus,** to aid removal of a cataract.

**Graft**   *Quick Reference:* Body component transplanted from one site to another.
*Advanced Reference:* Can involve tissue alone or entire organs. Autograft indicates when the donor is also the recipient, e.g. skin graft; *isograft* means a graft between identical individuals; *allograft*, between

dissimilar members of the same species; *xenograft*, between different species; orthotopic, a graft placed in the normal anatomical site; heterotopic, a graft placed in an anatomically abnormal site.

**Gram** *Quick Reference:* Unit of weight in the metric system.
*Advanced Reference:* 28 grams equate to 1 ounce.

**Gram's stain** *Quick Reference:* Method of staining bacteria.
*Advanced Reference:* The staining that enables the bacteria to be classified as either Gram negative or Gram positive.

**Granulation tissue** *Quick Reference:* Tissue formed at the site of a wound.
*Advanced Reference:* Composed mainly of small blood vessels and fibres. It is the first stage of healing.

**Granulocytes** *Quick Reference:* (gran-ulo-sites) Type of *white blood cell.*
*Advanced Reference:* White blood cells containing neutrophils, eosinophils and basophils.

**Granuloma** *Quick Reference:* Mass of granulation tissue.
*Advanced Reference:* Usually formed at the site of localised infection.

**Gravid** *Quick Reference:* Refers to pregnancy.
*Advanced Reference:* Gravid uterus. Primigravida refers to first pregnancy.

**Greenstick fracture** *Quick Reference:* Type of bone fracture.
*Advanced Reference:* Found in the long bones of children. The bone does not break completely, one side breaks while the other bends. This is due to the high level of connective tissue in children's bones as opposed to calcium and makes the bones more flexible.

**Grey matter** *Quick Reference:* Cellular tissue in the nervous system.
*Advanced Reference:* The brain and spinal cord contain two kinds of tissue, grey matter and white matter which are found in varying zones of these areas. In the spinal column, grey matter is gathered into a central column surrounded by white matter and in the brain is clumped into nuclei and over the surface of the *cerebrum* and *cerebellum.*

**Gridiron incision** *Quick Reference:* Incision used to access the appendix.
*Advanced Reference:* So named due to access being made via splitting the internal oblique and transverse muscles which have a 'gridiron' or 'mesh appearance'.

**Groin** *Quick Reference:* Area which includes the upper thigh and lower abdomen.
*Advanced Reference:* Used regularly but inaccurately in lay terms to indicate the genitalia.

**Grommet** *Quick Reference:* Tube inserted in the ear.

*Advanced Reference:* A grommet is a small plastic tube used to dry up glue ear. It is inserted into the ear drum creating a vent and a passage for drainage.

**Guedel** *Quick Reference:* (gudel) Oro-pharyngeal airway.

*Advanced Reference:* American anaesthetist known for introducing the oro-pharyngeal airway and devising the stages of anaesthesia.

**Guillotine:** *Quick Reference:* (gill-o-teen) Surgical instrument used in ear, nose and throat (ENT) surgery.

*Advanced Reference:* Instrument used for excision of the *tonsils*.

**Gullet** *Quick Reference:* The *oesophagus*.

*Advanced Reference:* Muscular tube connecting the throat to the *stomach*.

**Guns** *Quick Reference:* Slang term indicating mechanical stapling instruments.

*Advanced Reference:* Many are now available for anastomosing and suturing various organs and tissues. Their introduction has speeded up many surgical procedures.

**Gynaecology** *Quick Reference:* Medicine and surgery of the female reproductive system.

*Advanced Reference:* Gynaecology and *obstetrics* (the management of pregnancy) are counted as separate specialities though normally practised together by the one specialist.

**Gynaecomastia** *Quick Reference:* Abnormal enlargement of the male breasts.

*Advanced Reference:* May happen around the time of puberty due to hormonal imbalance. Can also be associated with over-activity of the thyroid, liver disease and conditions which are treated with oestrogens.

**Gypsum** *Quick Reference:* Plaster of Paris.

*Advanced Reference:* Calcium sulphate.

# H

**Haemaccel** *Quick Reference:* (hem-a-cel) Intravenous (IV) solution used as a plasma expander.

*Advanced Reference:* A gelatin solution with a high molecular weight (30,000) and therefore useful as a *plasma* expander. Due to its lengthy *shelf-life* is used in major accident packs where prolonged storage may be required. Known to produce hypersensitivity reactions so used with caution.

**Haematemesis** *Quick Reference:* (hem-a-tem-e-sis) Vomiting of blood.

*Advanced Reference:* Usually due to bleeding from the stomach. If dark in colour, can indicate that it has been in the stomach for a lengthy time and been partially digested by gastric secretions and often referred to as coffee-granule appearance.

**Haematocrit** *Quick Reference:* Total red cell volume (count).

*Advanced Reference:* Also referred to as packed cell volume (PCV) and expressed as a proportion of blood volume.

**Haematology** *Quick Reference:* (hem-a-tol-ogy) Indicates the blood.

*Advanced Reference:* The speciality that deals with the composition, function and disease of blood.

**Haematoma** *Quick Reference:* (hem-a-toe ma) A blood-filled swelling.

*Advanced Reference:* A swelling caused by bleeding into the tissues usually as the result of injury or after injection (intramuscular (*IM*), intravenous (*IV*), intra-arterial (*IA*), etc).

**Haematuria** *Quick Reference:* (hem-a-tur-ea) Blood in the urine.

*Advanced Reference:* Blood in the urine, usually a symptom of injury or disease to any part of the urinary tract. May also be witnessed short term following unconnected surgery of the pelvis and lower abdomen.

**Haemodialysis** *Quick Reference:* (hemo-di-al-a-sis) A form of renal dialysis.

*Advanced Reference:* One form of renal dialysis used in chronic renal failure via a *shunt* or atrioventricular (*AV*) *fistula*. See *renal dialysis*.

**Haemoglobin** *Quick Reference:* The red pigment of the blood carried by the red blood cells (erythrocyte). The abbreviation is Hb.

*Advanced Reference:* Composed of the protein globin and an iron compound, haem and is the means of transporting oxygen from the lungs to the rest of the body.

**Haemolysis**   *Quick Reference:* (hem-ol-y-sis) Breakdown of red blood cells.
*Advanced Reference:* The disintegration of red blood cells followed by the liberation of blood pigment into the circulation. Can occur in conditions of the new born, following heart valve surgery or due to parasites such as malaria or allergic reactions.

**Haemophilia**   *Quick Reference:* (hem-o-fil-ia) Blood disease involving deficiency of blood-clotting factors.
*Advanced Reference:* **Haemophilia** is an inherited disease affecting males but carried by females who remain unaffected. Haemophiliacs are unable to synthesise *factor VIII*. This absence produces prolonged and repeated *haemorrhage* which can be external or internal, the latter sometimes due to no obvious cause.

**Haemoptysis**   *Quick Reference:* (hem-op-te-sis) Coughing up or spitting of blood.
*Advanced Reference:* Can be due to bleeding within the mouth or nose or from the respiratory tract and lungs.

**Haemorrhage**   *Quick Reference:* (hem-or-age) Escape of blood from a vessel.
*Advanced Reference:* Haemorrhage or bleeding can be internal or external and from an artery, vein or capillary. In relation to theatre and surgery, there are three stages of bleeding: *primary*, which occurs at the time of operation; *reactionary*, which occurs within 24 h of injury or operation; *secondary*, occurs after 7–10 days post-operatively.

**Haemorrhoids**   *Quick Reference:* (hem-a-roids) Commonly referred to as piles.
*Advanced Reference:* **Varicose veins** found at the junction of the rectum and anal canal. Can be internal or external to the anal sphincter. Causes include constipation and uterine pressure during pregnancy.

**Halcion**   *Quick Reference:* (hal-see-on) Tranquilliser and hypnotic.
*Advanced Reference:* A preparation of the **benzodiazepine** triazolam used primarily to treat insomnia.

**Half-life**   *Quick Reference:* Time taken for a substance (e.g. radioactive, pharmaceutical) to fall or reduce to half its original value.
*Advanced Reference:* With regard to pharmacy, it is a measure of how long it takes for 50% of a drug to be excreted.

**Hallux**   *Quick Reference:* Indicating the big toe.
*Advanced Reference:* Hallux valgus refers to a bunion found on the big toe and removed surgically if causing problems. Usually due to the wearing of tight fitting shoes.

**Halothane**   *Quick Reference:* A volatile inhalational anaesthetic.

*Advanced Reference:* The commonly used trade name is *fluothane*. As with all volatile agents, it is colour coded (red) and delivered via an agent-specific vaporiser. Said to be non-irritant and does not cause post-operative nausea and vomiting (PONV); however, it has a disadvantage that repeated administration can cause liver damage.

**Hard palate**   *Quick Reference:* Bony portion of the roof of the mouth.

*Advanced Reference:* It is continuous posteriorly with the soft palate and bounded anteriorly and laterally by the gums.

**Harelip**   *Quick Reference:* (hair-lip) Congenital defect affecting the lip.

*Advanced Reference:* A failure of the two halves of the upper lip to join. Harelip is often associated with *cleft palate* which is a failure of the two sides of the palate to fuse together.

**Harness**   *Quick Reference:* Device for holding a face mask or airway equipment in place.

*Advanced Reference:* There are a number of different designs for holding the mask; e.g. Clausen, Connell, three-tailed and the Hudson which are used in such specialities as dental surgery, etc. and designed to fix the endotracheal (ET) tube and connections to the forehead.

**Hartmanns (solution)**   *Quick Reference:* An isotonic IV solution.

*Advanced Reference:* Used for general fluid replacement. It has a composition similar to plasma. Also referred to as *lactated ringers* solution and balanced salt solutions.

**HASAWA**   *Quick Reference:* Health and Safety at Work Act. UK legislation covering safety and health in the workplace, i.e. to protect employees while at work.

*Advanced Reference:* It was introduced in 1974 (replacing or incorporating existing laws, etc.) with the aim of providing a safe place of work and safe working conditions. An enabling act allowing additions and updates as and when necessary without again going through the full parliamentary process, e.g. control of substances hazardous to health (COSHH), manual handling regs, etc.

**Haversian canal**   *Quick Reference:* Longitudinal canal in bone tissue.

*Advanced Reference:* Carries blood vessels, nerves and in some instances lymph vessels.

**H$_2$-blocking drugs**   *Quick Reference:* Group of drugs that inhibit the manufacture of hydrochloric acid (HCl) in the stomach.

*Advanced Reference:* They actually work by inhibiting the receptors involved in the acid production. Used to reduce gastric acid prior to induction of anaesthesia in an effort to limit the possibility of *Mendelson's syndrome* (should aspiration occur), cimetidine is a common example.

Operating Department Practice A–Z

**Headlight**   *Quick Reference:* Operating light worn by the surgeon.

*Advanced Reference:* Popular with most specialities. Usually of *fibre-optic* design and attaches to a static light source. It is worn by the surgeon to supplement the operating lights and can focus on a particular area which might otherwise prevent illumination difficulties.

**Head-ring**   *Quick Reference:* Patient head support used during surgery.

*Advanced Reference:* Made of sponge and covered with black rubber or as a clear gel version; it is used when a pillow may be obstructive or as a means of stabilising the head position as in dental surgery.

**Health care assistant**   *Quick Reference:* Abbreviated as HCA; hospital support worker.

*Advanced reference:* Support worker with a role developed from that of orderly and auxiliary nurse. Most hospitals and the care home sectors introduced formal training for this group utilising the National Vocational Qualifications (NVQ) training system.

**Heart block**   *Quick Reference:* Interruption to the conducting channels of the heart.

*Advanced Reference:* Generally an interruption in conduction between the atria and ventricles due to fibrosis, lesion, etc. Seen as 1st-, 2nd- and 3rd-degree block, indicating level (bundle of His) affected and severity, causing significant electrocardiographical (ECG) changes. Treatment depends on degree and symptoms. With complete block a pacemaker is fitted.

**Heartburn**   *Quick Reference:* Burning pain felt behind the sternum.

*Advanced Reference:* Also known as pyrosis. A symptom of dyspepsia and *reflux* where gastric acid enters the oesophagus and mouth causing a burning sensation. Can be due to such conditions as *hiatus hernia.* Relieved by alkali preparations.

**Heart failure**   *Quick Reference:* When the heart loses its ability to produce sufficient output.

*Advanced Reference:* Can be acute or chronic and affect either right or left side of the heart. Dependent on side or site can produce many signs and symptoms including breathlessness and oedema (of lungs, ankles, etc.).

Also referred to as *cardiac failure.* It does not really indicate complete failure but that the heart does not function as effectively as it may.

**Heart–lung machine**   *Quick Reference:* Used primarily during open heart surgery.

*Advanced Reference:* Consists basically of a pump and an oxygenator. Takes over (bypasses) the function of the heart and lungs during open heart surgery by diverting the blood out via the venous system through the oxygenator and returns it to the arterial circulation.

**Heat loss**   *Quick Reference:* Usually refers to patient's heat loss while within the peri-operative period.

*Advanced Reference:* Most significant in the intra-operative phase during surgery. Patients lose heat by conduction, convection, radiation as well as via evaporation. A number of heat-loss preventing methods are employed including increased room temperature, additional clothing and coverings, warming of infused fluids, various designs of intra-operative under and over blankets, which utilise warm-air, electric elements and water heating combined with ripple effect for skin pressure protection.

**Heel (pad)**   *Quick Reference:* Pad placed under the heels during surgery.

*Advanced Reference:* Intended to relieve pressure on the calves and blood vessels when patient is in the *supine* position in an attempt to avoid pressure sores and deep vein thrombosis (*DVT*).

**Hegar's (dilators)**   *Quick Reference:* (ha-gars) Gynaecological dilator.

*Advanced Reference:* Set of graduated dilators used in *gynaecology* during dilatation and curettage (D&C), evacuation of retained products of conception (EVAC) of *uterus*, etc. to dilate the cervix, etc.

**Heidbrink (valve)**   *Quick Reference:* (hide-brink) Pressure-limiting valve.

*Advanced Reference:* An adjustable pressure-limiting valve found in a number of anaesthetic circuits, namely **Waters, Magill**, etc.

**Heimlich (manoeuvre)**   *Quick Reference:* (hime-lick) Emergency treatment for upper airway obstruction.

*Advanced Reference:* A manoeuvre taught in first aid and basic life support (BLS) intended to remove foreign body obstruction of the upper airway using compression of the upper abdomen. The rise in intrathoracic pressure creates a force which expels the cause of the obstruction.

**Helium**   *Quick Reference:* (He) Inert gas.

*Advanced Reference:* Combined helium–oxygen mixture is used as a method of delivering alveolar oxygen in patients with upper airway obstruction. Available as individual gas in brown cylinders or in a mixture with 21% oxygen in brown-bodied cylinders with brown and white shoulder.

**Hemi-arthroplasty**   *Quick Reference:* Replacement of half of hip joint.

*Advanced Reference:* **Arthroplasty** is the operative reconstruction of a joint due to injury or disease. With reference to the hip joint, can be total replacement or hemi. The latter involves replacement of the head of femur with a prosthesis made of inert material.

**Hemicolectomy**   *Quick Reference:* Surgical removal of a portion (approximately half) of the colon.

*Advanced Reference:* Also referred to as 'partial colectomy'. Involves removal of ascending and portion of transverse colon. Usual to have a transverse colostomy created following the procedure.

**Hemiplegia**   *Quick Reference:* (hemi-pleeg-ia) Half, paralysis of one side of the body.

*Advanced reference:* One-sided paralysis of the body, sometimes following cerebrovascular accident (CVA) when the opposite side has been injured. Person affected is referred to as a hemiplegic.

**Heparin**   *Quick Reference:* (hep-a-rin) An anticoagulant.

*Advanced Reference:* A naturally occurring anticoagulant manufactured in the liver. Used for general anticoagulant therapy and to prevent thrombosis and embolism. Has an immediate effect with a duration of action of 4–6 h. Antagonised by ***protamine*** and naturally in the body by the enzyme *heparinase* by preventing the action of thrombin on ***fibrinogen***.

**Hepatitis**   *Quick Reference:* Inflammation of the liver.

*Advanced Reference:* Mainly seen as type A (viral or infective), B (serum) and C, previously referred to as non-A and non-B. Due to differing causes: A viral through food or water(type A), blood-borne infection (type B), via blood (type C), etc. Sometimes recorded as acute or chronic. There are further strains referred to as D and E. Both active and passive immunity can be attained via injection.

**Hep-flush**   *Quick Reference:* Proprietary anticoagulant.

*Advanced Reference:* Contains ***heparin*** and used to wash and rinse the interior of catheters and cannulae, and other forms of tubing to ensure that they remain unobstructed by preventing clotting. Available also as *hepsal*.

**Hermaphrodite**   *Quick Reference:* (herm-af-ro-dite) Condition in which both male and female sex organs are present.

*Advanced Reference:* Hermaphrodites have the primary sex organs (ovaries and testes) of one sex but many secondary characters of the other.

**Herniorrhaphy**   *Quick Reference:* (her-nee-or-afi) Repair of *hernia* or rupture.

*Advanced Reference:* Operation to repair a hernia by reinforcing the weakened area with patient's own tissues or synthetic material, e.g. mesh.

**Heroin**   *Quick Reference:* A narcotic analgesic.

*Advanced Reference:* Alternative name is diamorphine. A powerful synthetic derivative of ***morphine*** prohibited in the US but prescribed in the UK mainly for intractable pain and palliative care. With reference to theatres, seen as an additive with spinal and epidural drugs.

**Herpes zoster**   *Quick Reference:* Shingles.

*Advanced Reference:* A virus also related to cause of chickenpox. Affects nerve routes causing pain and redness over site.

**Hespan**   *Quick Reference:* IV plasma expander, proprietary form of hetastarch. Also known as *pentaspan*.

*Advanced Reference:* A colloid solution presented in 6% strength, used for volume expansion. Has a high molecular weight (450,000) and is longer lasting than many alternative plasma expanders. Approximates in many aspects to human albumin.

**Hg**    *Quick Reference:* Symbol used to indicate mercury.
*Advanced Reference:* Witnessed in theatre environment with blood pressure (BP) readings; e.g. mmHg.

**Hiatus**    *Quick Reference:* (hi-a-tus) A space or opening.
*Advanced Reference:* Meaning half, in relation to theatres; seen as *hiatus hernia* where the stomach protrudes through the cardiac sphincter.

**Hiatus hernia**    *Quick Reference:* Protrusion of the upper part of the stomach through the oesophageal opening in the diaphragm.
*Advanced Reference:* Leads to escape of gastric acid into the oesophagus causing pain and heartburn. Worse after a heavy meal or when lying flat. If symptoms become severe can be corrected by surgery.

**Hibidil**    *Quick Reference:* Proprietary skin disinfectant.
*Advanced Reference:* Used also to treat wounds and burns. Produced in the form of a solution in sachets. It is a preparation of *chlorhexidine* gluconate.

**Hibiscrub**    *Quick Reference:* Proprietary disinfectant hand wash.
*Advanced Reference:* Used during the scrub-up prior to surgery. Is a preparation of *chlorhexidine* gluconate in a surfactant liquid, such as a detergent.

**Hibisol**    *Quick Reference:* Proprietary disinfectant used to treat minor wounds and burns of the skin.
*Advanced Reference:* It is a preparation of chlorhexidine gluconate in isopropyl alcohol together with emollients.

**Hibitane**    *Quick Reference:* (hib-i-tane). Form of disinfectant based on *chlorhexidine* solution.
*Advanced Reference:* A broad usage disinfectant derived from chlorhexidine solution and alternative chlorhexidine salts. Available as powder, creams, compounds and solutions, and for both internal and external use.

**Hiccup**    *Quick Reference:* (hic-up) Involuntary inspiratory spasm involving the muscles of respiration.
*Advanced Reference:* Also spelt hiccough (hic-cup). In hiccup there is a spasmodic contraction of the diaphragm and other respiratory organs followed by sudden closure of the vocal cords producing a characteristic sound.

**Hidrosis**    *Quick Reference:* To sweat.
*Advanced Reference:* Indicates the secretion of sweat.

**Hilum**    *Quick Reference:* (hi-lum) Point of attachment or entry.

*Advanced Reference:* A notch or hollow situated on the surface of an organ where blood vessels, nerves, etc. enter or leave. The renal hilum at the pelvis of the kidney.

**Hirschsprungs** *Quick Reference:* (hairs-sh-prungs) Congenital disease involving abnormal enlargement of the colon.

*Advanced Reference:* Congenital megacolon, involves a narrowed segment of bowel in the pelvic colon, causing a partial obstruction to the normal passage of faeces into the rectum resulting in dilatation of the bowel above the narrowing. This narrowing is a failure of nerve cell development in the affected area. Technically termed as *aganglionic megacolon*.

**Hirudoid** *Quick Reference:* Proprietary vasodilator and anticoagulant.

*Advanced Reference:* Intended to improve circulation in conditions such as *varicose veins*, bruising, etc. Available as a cream or gel for topical application. Its active constituent is a derivative of *heparin*.

**Hist(o)-** *Quick Reference:* Prefix denoting tissue.

*Advanced Reference:* Also referred to as his- and histo-; all denote tissue; e.g. hist-*pathology*, study of the changes in tissue due to disease.

**Histamine** *Quick Reference:* (hist-a-meen) A naturally occurring chemical in body tissues.

*Advanced Reference:* Released when tissues are injured causing a reaction in muscle and blood vessels. Sudden release due to reaction or sensitivity is witnessed as redness of skin (*urticaria*) and can lead to *anaphylaxis*.

**HME** *Quick Reference:* Heat and moisture exchanger.

*Advanced Reference:* Device placed within the patient anaesthetic circuitry designed to provide humidification using the patients own exhaled moisture and usually incorporates a bacterial filter.

**Hodgkin's disease** *Quick Reference:* Disorder of the lymph nodes and spleen.

*Advanced Reference:* May also affect the bone marrow and other areas involved in the defence against infection. Causes cell proliferation and swelling combined with fever and general sickness while lowering resistance.

**Hoffman prism** *Quick Reference:* Intubation aid.

*Advanced Reference:* A prism that slots onto the laryngoscope blade to aid visualisation during intubation.

**Holistic** *Quick Reference:* Indicates an overall approach to patient care.

*Advanced Reference:* An holistic approach to care involves not only attending to the current disease but also the entire physical, psychological and social factors affecting the patient.

**Homoeostasis**   *Quick Reference:* (home-eo-staysis) Process by which the internal body systems remain within normal limits despite changes in the external environment.

    *Advanced Reference:* Refers to the maintenance and function of the body's physiological state and keeping within normal limits. Mainly includes temperature, acid–base balance, BP, etc.

**Hormone**   *Quick Reference:* (hor-mone) A chemical (messenger) secreted into the bloodstream by an endocrine gland.

    *Advanced Reference:* A chemical released into the bloodstream by one organ (endocrine ductless gland) and has an effect on the function of other organs and tissues within the body.

**Horseshoe**   *Quick Reference:* Patient head support used during surgery.

    *Advanced Reference:* Horseshoe-shaped head rest more suitable for use when the patient is in the head-down position. Unlike the head-ring, the gap in the horseshoe allows a space for ET tube, tubing or as a gap to avoid eye pressure, etc. Made of sponge covered with black rubber or clear gel versions.

**Hotline**   *Quick Reference:* IV fluid warmer.

    *Advanced Reference:* Brand name for a fluid warmer. As fluid passes through it is warmed. Assists in offsetting temperature loss during surgical procedures.

**Hudson head harness**   *Quick Reference:* Device used to secure/fix *ET tube* in place.

    *Advanced Reference:* Harness that fits around forehead and secures ET tube and circuit in, e.g. dental surgery.

**Human actrapid**   *Quick Reference:* Proprietary preparation of synthesised neutral human insulin.

    *Advanced Reference:* Used to treat and maintain diabetic patients. Produced in vials for injection and cartridges for use with a special injector.

**Human albumin solution (HAS)**   *Quick Reference:* IV solution used as a plasma expander.

    *Advanced Reference:* HAS is a form of *pasteurised* plasma heated to 60°C and used as a *plasma expander*.

**Hyalase**   *Quick Reference:* (hi-al-ase) Form of hyaluronidase.

    *Advanced Reference:* Used to increase the permeability of subcutaneous tissue or muscles into which drugs can be injected. Commonly used when injected drugs have 'tissued' (*extravasated*). Available as a powder for reconstitution.

**Hyaline**   *Quick Reference:* Substance that is clear or glass like.

    *Advanced Reference:* Hyaline cartilage is a type of elastic connective tissue composed of special cells in a translucent matrix.

**Hydatid (disease)**   *Quick Reference:* (hi-dat-id) Infection with a type of tapeworm.

*Advanced Reference:* The disease usually forms cysts mainly in the liver and lungs which need to be removed surgically. The cysts are formed by the larvae of the tapeworm and passed on from dogs to other animals, e.g. sheep or via contact. The *cysts* may become infected or burst and set off an anaphylactic reaction.

**Hydralazine**   *Quick Reference:* Vasodilator.

*Advanced Reference:* Used for treatment of both acute and chronic hypertension. Alternative name is apresoline. Can be administered orally or IV. Used for treatment of both acute and chronic *hypertension*.

**Hydration**   *Quick Reference:* A chemical process in which water is added without disrupting the rest of the molecule.

*Advanced Reference:* Refers to the amount (adequate or otherwise) of water in the intracellular and extracellular compartments of the body. To *hydrate* is to provide fluid and to *rehydrate* is to replace fluid.

**Hydrocele**   *Quick Reference:* (hydro-seal) Collection of fluid surrounding the testicle.

*Advanced Reference:* The fluid collects in the sac (tunica vaginalis). Occurs with no obvious cause. Treatment can be through aspiration but as incidence of re-occurrence is high, surgery for removal of the sac is the normal course of treatment.

**Hydrocephalus**   *Quick Reference:* (hydro-cef-alus) Accumulation of cerebrospinal fluid (CSF) in the ventricles of the brain.

*Advanced Reference:* Caused by obstruction through the ventricles and into the *arachnoid* space or failure of absorption. Causes include *meningitis, adhesions.*

**Hydrochloric acid**   *Quick Reference:* HCl, found in normal gastric juices in dilute form.

*Advanced Reference:* Formed from a solution of hydrogen gas and water.

**Hydrocortisone**   *Quick Reference:* Hormone secreted from the adrenal cortex.

*Advanced Reference:* A corticosteroid used for replacement therapy and suppression of allergic and inflammatory reactions.

**Hydrogen**   *Quick Reference:* Chemical symbol H.

*Advanced Reference:* A gaseous element, colourless, odourless and highly inflammable. Combines with oxygen to form water ($H_2O$). ***Hydrogen ion concentration*** indicates the acidity or alkalinity (***pH***) of a solution.

**Hydrogen peroxide**   *Quick Reference:* Wound cleaning fluid.

*Advanced Reference:* A mild disinfecting and mainly cleaning fluid used usually in a 6% solution for flushing wounds of debris and dressing residue. Its cleaning action is due to liberation of oxygen as it decomposes into water and oxygen as tissue contact is made.

**Hydrogen ion concentration**   *Quick Reference:* Related to pH (acid/alkali) status.

*Advanced Reference:* The number of hydrogen ions in a solution is a measure of the acidity of the solution.

**Hydrometer**   *Quick Reference:* A calibrated hollow glass device used for measuring the *specific gravity* or *density* of a liquid.

*Advanced Reference:* Works by comparing its weight with that of an equal volume of water.

**Hydronephrosis**   *Quick Reference:* (hydro-nef-rosis) Distention of the renal pelvis.

*Advanced Reference:* Caused by obstruction to urine flow due to stones, tumour, narrowing of the **ureter** following tuberculosis (TB) or congenital reasons. Treatment depends on cause, but a kidney badly affected usually requires surgery with the aim of preserving as much as possible or removal if necessary.

**Hydrosalpinx**   *Quick Reference:* Abnormal condition of the fallopian tubes.

*Advanced Reference:* In this condition, the fallopian tubes become cystically enlarged and filled with clear fluid and is the result of infection which has sealed off the ends of the tubes.

**Hygrometer**   *Quick Reference:* (hi-grom-eter) Instrument for measuring the amount of moisture in the atmosphere.

*Advanced Reference:* In the context of theatres, measures the relative humidity, which is the amount of moisture present in the air compared to the amount which would saturate it at the same temperature. Too high (moist) or too low (dry), both have inherent hazards; 50–55% is regarded as safe and suitable for most theatre situations and comfort of staff.

**Hyoscine**   *Quick Reference:* (hio-seen) Alkaloid drug with hypnotic properties.

*Advanced Reference:* Obtained from *Belladonna*. An **anticholinergic** agent with similar properties to Atropine causing *sedation* and **tachycardia** and used as an alternative in premedication. Alternative name is buscopan.

**Hyper-**   *Quick Reference:* (hi-per) Above or too much.

*Advanced Reference:* A prefix indicating over or above the normal as in *hypertension*, high BP; *hyperglycaemia*, high blood sugar; *hyperpyrexia*, abnormally high body temperature; etc.

**Hyperbaric**   *Quick Reference:* (hi-per-bar-ic) A greater than normal pressure, weight or *specific gravity*.

*Advanced Reference:* In relation to theatres, hyperbaric (heavy) drugs are used during spinal analgesia. Also, hyperbaric oxygen chambers, when patient is referred for certain conditions, i.e. *gangrene.* The anaerobic organisms responsible are adversely affected by the presence of oxygen.

**Hyperplasia** *Quick Reference:* Increased production and growth of tissue.
*Advanced Reference:* The increase in the size of tissue or an organ due to enlargement of its cells rather than by multiplication.

**Hypertension** *Quick Reference:* High BP.
*Advanced Reference:* May be a disease in its own right or symptoms of a recognised disease. These may include *renal* hypertension, *pulmonary* hypertension and *malignant* hypertension. Continued hypertension can eventually lead to damage in other areas, such as stroke and kidney damage.

**Hyperthermia** *Quick Reference:* (hi-per-therm-ea) Usually indicates a core body temperature greater than 40°C.
*Advanced Reference:* Can be accidental, in cases such as *malignant hyperpyrexia* or induced therapeutically in the treatment of, e.g. malignant disease.

**Hypertonic** *Quick Reference:* A solution with a higher osmotic pressure than the other.
*Advanced Reference:* Hypertonic saline has a higher osmotic pressure than normal saline. *Mannitol* is another example of a hypertonic solution. The opposite being *hypotonic,* a fluid with a lower osmotic pressure than the other.

**Hypertrophy** *Quick Reference:* (hi-per-troffy) Excessive or increased growth of tissue.
*Advanced Reference:* The increase in the size of tissue or organ due to enlargement of its cells rather than by cell multiplication.

**Hypnotic** *Quick Reference:* (hip-not-ic) Drug used to promote sleep.
*Advanced Reference:* Related in action to sedatives and narcotics, differences being in terms of potency and effect. *Benzodiazepines* being the most widely used as hypnotics.

**Hypo-** *Quick Reference:* (hi-po) Prefix indicating below or too little.
*Advanced Reference:* Indicates below normal as in *hypotension,* low BP, *hypoglycaemia,* low blood sugar; *hypochondria,* below the ribs; etc.

**Hypochlorite** *Quick Reference:* (hi-po-clor-ite) Related to antiseptics and disinfectants.

*Advanced Reference:* A salt of hypochlorous acid. These salts have both antiseptic and disinfectant properties, and when decomposed yield active chlorine. *Milton* is an example.

**Hypochondrium** *Quick Reference:* (hi-po-con-dri-um) Area of the abdomen covered by the cartilage of the lower ribs.

*Advanced Reference:* The upper lateral parts of the abdomen lying to the right and left of the *epigastric* region.

**Hypodermic** *Quick Reference:* (hi-po-der-mic) Below or under the skin.

*Advanced Reference:* The term usually refers to *subcutaneous* injections and also applied to indicate the needle and syringe used for the procedure.

**Hypoglycaemia** *Quick Reference:* (hi-po-gli-cem-ia) Deficiency of sugar in the blood.

*Advanced Reference:* The usual cause is an imbalance between sugar levels and available insulin. The excess of insulin uses up glucose from the blood by increased combustion. In diabetics, this can arise from too much insulin or wrong diet. Can also be due to overactivity. Symptoms include perspiration, excitement, delirium and eventually coma.

**Hyponatraemia** *Quick Reference:* (hi-po-nat-rem-ia) Low level of sodium in the blood.

*Advanced Reference:* A blood-sodium level away from the normal range of 135–150 mmol/l. Can be due to excessive diarrhoea and vomiting, sweating, burns and some renal conditions. Treatment is usually with 0.9% saline but in severe cases *hypertonic saline* may be used. In theatres seen as trans-urethral resection (TUR) syndrome (water intoxication) caused by irrigation of the bladder, even with 1.5% **glycine** during trans-urethral resection of the prostate (TURP) when water enters the open prostatic veins resulting in a number of symptoms seen mainly in recovery, e.g. restlessness, confusion, abdominal pain, shortness of breath and possibly cardiac arrest.

**Hypospadias** *Quick Reference:* (hi-po-spade-ius) Congenital malformation of the penis.

*Advanced Reference:* The **genital** folds fail to unite in the midline and the opening of the urethra may be found anywhere on the undersurface of the penis or even in the *perineum*.

**Hypotensive anaesthesia** *Quick Reference:* Techniques used for lowering BP during anaesthesia.

*Advanced Reference:* The aim is to lower BP and so improve operating conditions for the surgeon. Common in ear, nose and throat (ENT) surgery (inner ear surgery). May involve a number of drugs which directly lower BP or combinations of anaesthetic drugs which have this effect. Patient positioning (head-up/down) is also used for some procedures and spinal/epidural anaesthesia can be utilised for the same purpose.

**Hypothalamus**   *Quick Reference:* Part of the brain that lies at the base, below the third ventricle and below the thalamus.

*Advanced Reference:* It controls the vegetative functions, such as body temperature, appetite, BP, fluid balance and sleep.

**Hypothermia**   *Quick Reference:* (hi-po-thermia) A lowering of body temperature.

*Advanced Reference:* Body temperature below the normal range. Can be accidental, which occurs if normal homeostasis fails and heat loss exceeds heat production, or deliberately induced as for surgery in order to slow metabolism and the requirement for oxygen. Measured sometimes as mild, moderate and severe (deep). Said to become a clinical problem when the core temperature falls below 36°C.

**Hypovolaemia**   *Quick Reference:* (hi-po-vol-eemia) Reduced quantity of blood.

*Advanced Reference:* Indicates a reduction in circulating blood volume usually due to bleeding (external or internal) causing a drop in BP and leading to hypovolaemic shock.

**Hypoxia**   *Quick Reference:* Deficiency of oxygen in the tissues.

*Advanced Reference:* Related to *anoxia* in which tissues receive inadequate or literally no oxygen. Also *hypoxia*. All recognised clinically by the presence of *cyanosis*.

**Hysterectomy**   *Quick Reference:* Surgical removal of the uterus.

*Advanced Reference:* Removal of the *uterus*; either via abdomen or vagina. Performed for a variety of reasons including cancer, bleeding, etc. The abdominal approach can involve various degrees of removal, including sub-total, total, *pan* and *Wertheims*, which is the removal of uterus, tubes, ovaries, upper part of vagina plus pelvic lymph glands.

**Hysterogram**   *Quick Reference:* (his-ter-o-gram) *X-ray* examination of the *uterus* and *fallopian* tubes.

*Advanced Reference:* Also termed hysterosalpingogram and hysterosalpingography. Involves injection of a contrast medium for X-ray of the uterus and fallopian tubes mostly to determine patency.

**Hysteroscopy**   *Quick Reference:* Inspection of the uterus through a rigid telescope.

*Advanced Reference:* A gynaecological procedure that is used as a diagnostic tool to inspect the endometrial lining of the uterus. Great care must be taken to initially establish the depth (size of the uterus) by using a uterine sound. Potential risk is to insert the telescope too far and puncture the fundus of the uterus.

**Hysterotomy**   *Quick Reference:* Opening into the uterus.

*Advanced Reference:* Usually involves surgical opening into the uterus in order to remove a *foetus*.

**Hyoid (bone)**   *Quick Reference:* (hi-oid) Small bone to which the tongue is attached.

*Advanced Reference:* Small U-shaped bone in the neck situated below the jaw and above the *larynx* to which many surrounding muscles are attached.

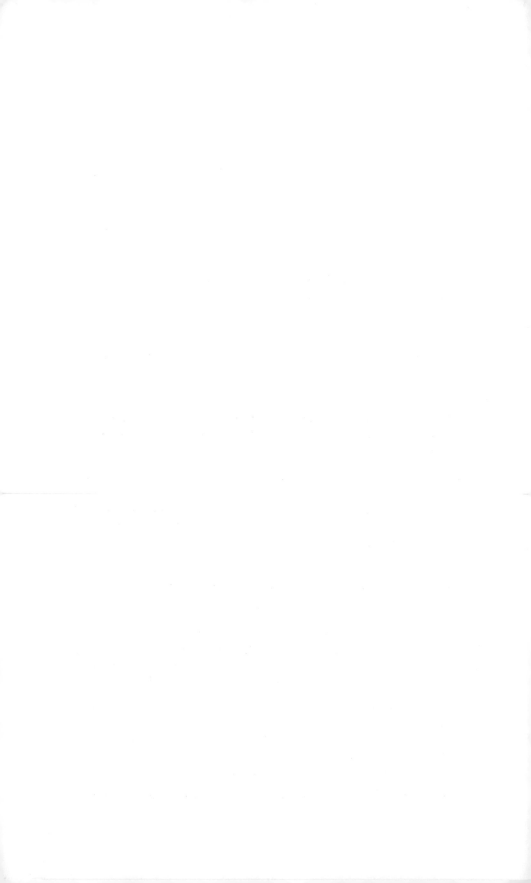

**Iatrogenic**   *Quick Reference:* Caused by treatment or diagnosis.
*Advanced Reference:* A disorder caused by physician or during the course of treatment within a health care facility.

**Idiopathic**   *Quick Reference:* Of unknown causation.
*Advanced Reference:* A term applied to diseases when their cause is unknown or of spontaneous origin.

**I : E ratio**   *Quick Reference:* Inspiratory : expiratory ratio.
*Advanced Reference:* Refers to the ratio between inspiration and expiration usually when a patient is being mechanically ventilated. This is normally 1 : 2.

**Ileostomy**   *Quick Reference:* An artificial opening between the ileum and the exterior (abdominal wall).
*Advanced Reference:* Created surgically in the right lower abdominal wall when the colon (large bowel) has been removed. Due to such causes as *ulcerative colitis*.

**Ileum**   *Quick Reference:* A section of the small intestine.
*Advanced Reference:* Involves the last three-fifths of the small intestine between the jejunum above and the caecum below.

**Ileus**   *Quick Reference:* An obstruction of the intestine.
*Advanced Reference:* Intestinal obstruction due to a number of causes including obliteration of the lumen by a tumour, strangulation, twisting or paralysis. Signs include abdominal distention and vomiting.

**Iliac crest**   *Quick Reference:* Iliac is a suffix indicating the ilium. Crest is a ridge or protuberance, usually of a bone.
*Advanced Reference:* The area of the upper elevated margins of the ilium but refers to the external bony prominence of the outer pelvis felt under the skin and used regularly as landmarks for surgery, etc.

**Image intensifier**   *Quick Reference:* Also referred to as the 'C-arm'. A mobile X-ray machine.

I

*Advanced Reference:* Used in theatres for situations other than the need for just X-ray pictures, i.e. orthopaedics being the most common. It amplifies the fluoroscopic optical image and projects it on to a television screen. The shape enables access to difficult areas during surgery and can facilitate screening from anterior to lateral positions as well as being able to produce traditional X-ray films.

**Immobilisation**   *Quick Reference:* Fixation of a body part.
*Advanced Reference:* Indicates the fixation of a body part so that it cannot move during or after surgery, as with the setting of a fracture.

**Immunity**   *Quick Reference:* The process in the body of identifying and getting rid of invading organisms and foreign matter.
*Advanced Reference:* The word indicates the resistance to subsequent attacks conferred by one attack of an infectious disease or by a simulated attack such as vaccination (immunisation). Immunology is the study of immunity and the body's defence system.

**Immunosuppressants**   *Quick Reference:* Drugs used to inhibit the body's resistance to the presence of foreign bodies. Cyclosporin is an example.
*Advanced Reference:* Such drugs may be used to suppress tissue rejection following transplantation or donor grafting but then creates the risk of unopposed infection.

**Impedance**   *Quick Reference:* It is the resistance of alternating current (AC) flow in an electrical circuit.
*Advanced Reference:* The unit of impedance is the *ohm*. Involves resistors and capacitors. *Conductors* are substances with low impedance and those with high impedance are known as *insulators*.

**Implant**   *Quick Reference:* To set into (something).
*Advanced Reference:* Term often used to indicate a device set into the body. Examples are implantation of a joint, embryo implant into the uterus as in assisted fertility or radiological implant.

**Imuran**   *Quick Reference:* Proprietary preparation of the cytotoxic drug *azathioprine*.
*Advanced Reference:* Used to suppress tissue rejection following donor grafting or transplant surgery.

**Incidence**   *Quick Reference:* Number of times an event occurs.
*Advanced Reference:* In epidemiology the number of new cases in a particular period.

**Incident reporting**   *Quick Reference:* Written or verbal reporting of an event or series of occurrences.
*Advanced Reference:* Refers to any event that is inconsistent with desired patient outcomes or routines within a health care setting.

**Incision**   *Quick Reference:* A surgical cut into the body tissue using a scalpel and blade.

*Advanced Reference:* An incision is made into or over an operative site with the intention of providing access to underlying structures and organs etc. Some of the most common abdominal incisions are: Midline & Paramedian for e.g. *laparotomy*, McBurney (*Grid-Iron*) for *Appendicectomy*; Sub-costal (Kochers) for *Cholecystectomy; Pfannenstiel* for *Caesarean Section, Hysterectomy.*

**Incompatibility**   *Quick Reference:* Unable to co-exist.

*Advanced Reference:* In relation to tissue transplantation, there may be rejection because donor and recipient antibodies are incompatible.

**Incontinence**   *Quick Reference:* Inability to control bladder or bowel.

*Advanced Reference:* Due to diseases of the nervous system and particularly in women, weakness of the muscles of the pelvic floor (stress incontinence). When control of both bladder and bowel is lost it is termed double incontinence.

**Increment**   *Quick Reference:* To deliver small amounts of a total. To increase.

*Advanced Reference:* Used to describe the ***intermittent*** administration of drugs by small amounts (increments).

**Incubator**   *Quick Reference:* Apparatus used to provide a controlled environment.

*Advanced Reference:* Involves the control of light, temperature, moisture, oxygen, etc., as used in laboratory cultivation of micro-organisms and the newborn.

**Indicator tape**   *Quick Reference:* Refers to a number of colour-change tapes used in various sterilisation processes.

*Advanced Reference:* The most commonly used are those in steam and ethylene oxide sterilisation processes. They indicate exposure to the process rather than actual sterilisation by colour change.

**Indigo-carmine**   *Quick Reference:* A dye used usually in a 0.4% solution.

*Advanced Reference:* Given intravenously (IV) for testing renal function and for identifying vessels during certain types of surgery, i.e. ***thyroid***; also used for confirming patency of ***fallopian tubes*** during ***hysterogram.***

**Induce**   *Quick Reference:* To stimulate the start of an activity.

*Advanced Reference:* It means to induce *labour*, to induce an *abortion*. An enzyme induces a metabolic activity.

**Induction**   *Quick Reference:* To begin or set in motion.

*Advanced Reference:* Used commonly with reference to anaesthesia or labour, i.e. to induce labour or anaesthesia.

**Inert**   *Quick Reference:* Without any (chemical) action or reaction. Inert gases are present in air but appear to play no part in respiration.

*Advanced Reference:* Used in relation to implants and prosthesis made of 'inert' materials which indicates that they will cause no or little biological reaction, e.g. titanium joints, silicone catheters, etc.

**Infarct (ion)**   *Quick Reference:* Blockage of a blood vessel on which part of an organ depends.

*Advanced Reference:* Infarction can lead to death and scarring of affected tissue with the segment lost being called an infarct. Found commonly in cardiac, mesenteric, tissue.

**Infiltration**   *Quick Reference:* Indicates the injection of local anaesthetic (LA) into the subcutaneous and intradermal tissue.

*Advanced Reference:* Used for minor surgery solely as pain relief, for infiltration of the surgical incision to provide post-operative pain relief as well as a means of creating a bloodless field when the LA contains a vaso-constrictor such as adrenaline.

**Inflammation**   *Quick Reference:* The local reaction of the body to damage caused by infection or injury.

*Advanced Reference:* Inflammation is the natural response to injury of almost any kind and is the first stage of healing. The classic signs are redness and swelling with heat and pain.

**Infrared**   *Quick Reference:* Electromagnetic radiation beyond the red end of the spectrum.

*Advanced Reference:* Infrared is comprised of long invisible rays which are used therapeutically in numerous forms, mainly to produce heat in tissues. Classified as *non-ionising* radiation.

**Infusion**   *Quick Reference:* Refers to the slow injection of fluids and/or medication.

*Advanced Reference:* The IV administration of fluids, usually with added drugs, under the influence of gravity, as opposed to a direct injection with a syringe.

**Inguinal**   *Quick Reference:* (in-gwi-nal) Of the groin.

*Advanced Reference:* The inguinal region comprises the fold in front of the hip joint where the muscles of the abdomen and thigh meet. The part of the abdomen surrounding the inguinal canal, a common site of hernia.

**Inhalation**   *Quick Reference:* Method of introducing drugs into the body via the lungs.

*Advanced Reference:* A number of methods are used, i.e. aerosol, spacer, nebuliser; in anaesthesia *vaporisers* are the common method of delivering volatile agents.

**Injection**   *Quick Reference:* The act of administering liquid into the body.

*Advanced Reference:* Carried out usually with a syringe and needle via many routes; IV, intramuscular, subcutaneous, intra-dermal, intra-osseous, etc.

**Inoculation** *Quick Reference:* Introduction of material, etc. into the tissues or culture medium.

*Advanced Reference:* In relation to tissues, inoculation usually indicates the introduction of a *vaccine* but with a culture medium involves the introduction of a micro-organism for propagation.

**Inoperable** *Quick Reference:* Term used with reference to surgery when a condition or disease has progressed too far and nothing further (surgically) can be done.

*Advanced Reference:* Most common example is when a procedure cannot continue or be attempted due spread of cancer.

**Inotropic** *Quick Reference:* Anything that effects the force of muscle contraction.

*Advanced Reference:* Usually applied to cardiac muscle. Drugs such as **beta-blockers** are said to be inotropic.

**Institute of Operating Theatre Technicians (IOTT)** *Quick Reference:* Forerunner of Association of Operating Department Practitioners (AODP).

*Advanced Reference:* Prior to AODP and BAODA (British Association of Operating Department Assistants) IOTT was the representative professional body/organisation.

**Insufflation** *Quick Reference:* To blow air, gas, powder down a tube.

*Advanced Reference:* Indicates the blowing of air, etc. down a tube or into a body cavity; e.g. insufflating **carbon dioxide** ($CO_2$) into the peritoneal cavity for **laparoscopy** or blowing gas through fallopian tubes to establish patency. An insufflator is used to deliver the gas, etc.

**Insulin** *Quick Reference:* A **hormone** found in the **pancreas**.

*Advanced Reference:* Insulin is released into the bloodstream where it promotes the uptake of glucose for use by the body cells. Without it, glucose is neither consumed as fuel nor adequately stored and accumulates in the blood.

**Intensive care** *Quick Reference:* Specialised hospital ward.

*Advanced Reference:* Specialised ward for patients requiring intensive care and treatment. In some instances also referred to as intensive therapy unit (ITU).

**Intercostal** *Quick Reference:* Indicates area between the ribs.

*Advanced Reference:* Used to describe the blood vessels, nerves and muscles lying between the ribs.

**Intercurrent** *Quick Reference:* Occurring during the progress of another.

I

*Advanced Reference:* Illness or condition arising in the course of another illness. Intercurrent disease.

**Intermittent**   *Quick Reference:* At intervals, rather than all at one time.

*Advanced Reference:* Used in relation to (i) *intermittent injection*, i.e. giving *increments* of a drug rather than one single dose; (ii) *intermittent pain*, i.e. pain that is not constant but comes and goes; (iii) *intermittent positive-pressure ventilation (IPPV)*, i.e. intermittent ventilation of the lungs.

**Intermittent claudication**   *Quick Reference:* Muscle pain that comes on after exercise.

*Advanced Reference:* Caused by arterial disease, usually affecting the calf muscles. Due to the muscles being starved of oxygen by the poor blood supply and therefore unable to get rid of waste products, e.g. *lactic acid.*

**Interstitial**   *Quick Reference:* Indicates the spaces between the tissues/cells.

*Advanced Reference:* As opposed to intercellular, it is the fluid in which body cells are bathed. Also, sometimes termed *background tissue*, which supports the active tissue of an organ.

**Intestinal bag**   *Quick Reference:* A surgical sundry used to hold the intestines during abdominal surgery.

*Advanced Reference:* The intestines are placed into a clear plastic bag to help prevent fluid and heat loss during surgery. Also the clear plastic allows the surgeon to observe the intestine for any colour changes.

**Intestine**   *Quick Reference:* The *alimentary* canal after it leaves the stomach.

*Advanced Reference:* Comprised of the *small intestine*, *duodenum*, *pylorus*, *jejunum*, *ileum* and *large intestine* which terminates at the *anus.*

**Intra-occular**   *Quick Reference:* Within the eyeball.

*Advanced Reference:* Indicates pressure inside the eye, as in glaucoma.

**Intra-osseus**   *Quick Reference:* Indicates into a bone.

*Advanced Reference:* An intra-osseus infusion is injection of fluids/blood, etc. into the bone marrow. Used in emergency situations when IV access is not possible. Also commonly used with children.

**Intrathecal**   *Quick Reference:* Within a sheath.

*Advanced Reference:* As with intrathecal injection, i.e. the injection of LAs into the spinal canal (spinal anaesthesia).

**Intubation**   *Quick Reference:* The introduction of a tube into the body.

*Advanced Reference:* The term most commonly refers to intubation of the trachea with an *endotracheal* (ET) tube.

**Intussusception**   *Quick Reference:* Condition in which part of the intestine telescopes into the next segment.

*Advanced Reference:* Most cases occur in infants but may be seen in adults. Examples are the large intestine *invaginating* into itself or the last part of the ileum *prolapsing* into the caecum. Can lead to obstruction which requires surgical intervention.

**Invaginate**   *Quick Reference:* To fold inwards.
*Advanced Reference:* This folding in can lead to the formation of a pouch, as with intussusception of the intestine.

**Iodine**   *Quick Reference:* A naturally occurring element.
*Advanced Reference:* In medicine, it is essential for the correct functioning of the *thyroid* gland and also used in solution as an effective *antiseptic*.

**Ionisation**   *Quick Reference:* Term used with reference to high-energy electromagnetic waves, such as X-rays and gamma rays.
*Advanced Reference:* Ionising radiations are so called because when they pass through matter they cause ionisation, whereby neutral atoms acquire a temporary electric charge. X-rays and gamma rays are examples of ionising radiation. Ionising radiation has penetrative powers whereas non-ionising does not. Ultraviolet and infrared are examples of non-ionising radiation.

**Ionise(ing)**   *Quick Reference:* With reference to radiation (ionising and non-ionising).
*Advanced Reference:* X-rays are the common example of ionising radiation. When ionising radiation passes through the body it can bring about changes in cells, etc.

**Iris**   *Quick Reference:* The coloured part of the eye.
*Advanced Reference:* Lies behind the *cornea* and is comprised of two muscle layers which alter the size of the pupil and so control the amount of light entering the eye. *Iritis* is inflammation of the iris and *iridectomy* is removal of part of the iris usually due to *glaucoma*.

**Iron**   *Quick Reference:* Naturally occurring metallic element.
*Advanced Reference:* Heamoglobin (Hb) is made up of an iron compound (haem). Iron-deficiency anaemia is a common type of anaemia.

**Irradiation**   *Quick Reference:* Exposure to radiation.
*Advanced Reference:* Usually refers to treatment by ionising radiation for cancer treatment.

**Irrigation**   *Quick Reference:* To supply a stream of water or other fluid.
*Advanced Reference:* The washing out of a cavity or wound by a stream of water or other fluid. Examples are *lavage* of a wound or bladder irrigation during or after surgery of the *prostate gland*.

**Ischaemia**   *Quick Reference:* (is-keem-ea) Inadequate blood supply to a part of the body.

*Advanced Reference:* May be due to spasm, disease of the blood vessels or failure of the general circulation. If prolonged, the affected tissue dies. A common example is myocardial ischaemia, which occurs when the heart muscle receives inadequate blood supply.

**Ischiorectal abscess** *Quick Reference:* (isio-rectal) An *abscess* occurring between the rectum and ischium (lower posterior part of the pelvis).
*Advanced Reference:* Normally involves pus formation in the connective tissue often resulting in anal *fistula*.

**Islets of Langerhans** *Quick Reference:* Specialised cells found within the pancreas.
*Advanced Reference:* A cluster of cells in the pancreas which produces *insulin* and *glucagon*, and are released directly into the circulation where they play a part in glucose metabolism.

**Isoflurane** *Quick Reference:* A volatile anaesthetic agent.
*Advanced Reference:* A colourless liquid that allows rapid induction and recovery from anaesthesia.

**Isograft** *Quick Reference:* Type of graft.
*Advanced Reference*: A *graft* or transplant carried out between identical individuals.

**Isolation** *Quick Reference:* Separation of an infective patient from others.
*Advanced Reference:* Usually involves an isolation ward or area with the intention of preventing the spread of infecting organisms. Also used for patients with a deficient *immune* system. The technique is called *barrier nursing*.

**Isoprenaline** *Quick Reference:* Cardiac stimulant closely related to *adrenaline*, e.g. saventrine.
*Advanced Reference:* Increases both the heart rate and force of contraction. May also be used in treating *bronchospasm*. Used to treat extremely slow heart rate. Sometimes referred to as a chemical pacemaker.

**Isopropyl** *Quick Reference:* $C_3H_8O$. Clear, colourless alcohol.
*Advanced Reference:* Used as a 70% solution for skin prepping and cleaning in theatres.

**Isotonic** *Quick Reference:* Refers to solutions which have the same osmotic pressure as plasma.
*Advanced Reference:* **Normal saline** (0.9% NaCl) is isotonic with *plasma*, this means that it will not draw fluid from tissues nor be absorbed into them. **Hypertonic** solutions will withdraw fluid from the tissues and *hypotonic* solutions will be drawn into them.

**Isotope** *Quick Reference:* A chemical element.

*Advanced Reference:* An isotope which has the same atomic number as another but a different atomic mass. It has the same number of protons in the nucleus but a different number of neutrons.

**IUCD** *Quick Reference:* Intrauterine contraceptive device. Device fitted to women to prevent pregnancy.

*Advanced Reference:* Usually made from plastic or metal and is inserted into the uterus.

**Ivor Lewis** *Quick Reference:* Oesophagectomy. Surgical procedure for tumours of the oesophagus.

*Advanced Reference:* Carried out for the treatment of growths in the upper third of the oesophagus.

**IVP** *Quick Reference:* Intravenous *pyelogram:* Radiological technique for demonstrating the outline and function of the kidneys, ureter and bladder.

*Advanced Reference:* Involves the IV injection of a radio-opaque dye and as this is excreted by the kidneys, *X-rays* are taken to ascertain outline, function, general malfunction or obstruction to flow.

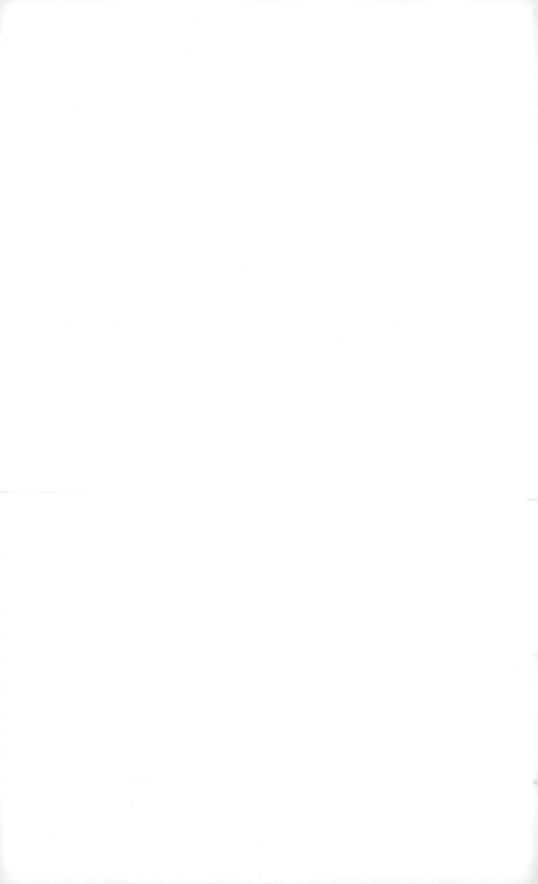

# J

**Jaboulay amputation**   *Quick Reference:* Also known as hindquarter amputation.

*Advanced Reference:* The amputation of the whole lower limb with corresponding iliac bone through the sacro-iliac joint. This is regarded as a mutilating operation and is usually performed because of a chondrosarcoma of the pelvis or upper femur.

**Jaboulay pyloroplasty**   *Quick Reference:* A side-to-side gastroduodenostomy.

*Advanced Reference:* This is performed when the pylorus and proximal duodenum are extensively scarred or indurated by peptic ulcer disease.

**Jack knife**   *Quick Reference:* Surgical operating position.

*Advanced Reference:* Involves the patient laying on their stomach with the hips flexed and knees bent at 90° and arms outstretched in front. Used for various spinal and rectal procedures.

**Jackscrew**   *Quick Reference:* A threaded screw.

*Advanced Reference:* A threaded device used in orthodontic appliances for the separation or approximation of teeth or jaw segments.

**Jackson Rees T-piece**   *Quick Reference:* A modification of the *Ayre's T-piece.*

*Advanced Reference:* Jackson Rees modification to an existing Ayre's T-piece within a paediatric breathing system to ensure that fresh gas flow (FGF) would remain separate from the exhaust gas. The modifications followed on from the *Jackson Rees T-tube.*

**Jackson Rees T-tube**   *Quick Reference:* Paediatric tube that incorporates a suction device.

*Advanced Reference:* FGF with flow across the intersection where the paediatric tube connected with the bar creating the famous T-shape. The top end of the paediatric tube had a removal bung inside. This could be withdrawn when there was a need to aspirate any secretions within the child lungs. The opposite end of the FGF flowing across the cross bar of the T-piece was an open-ended corrugated tubing for expired gas to escape under the direct positive pressure exerted by the patient. A passive scavenging system.

**Jacobs chuck**   *Quick Reference:* Holding jaws on a power drill used in orthopaedic surgery.

*Advanced Reference:* Jacobs chuck has three equal jaws that move in and out on an access to allow the insertion of drills or guide wires of all different sizes. Care should be taken with insertion that the drill or guide wire is central and proportionate on all three jaws. This can be achieved by inserting and turning the chuck key in each locating hole with the same number of turns.

**Jacques catheter**   *Quick Reference:* (jakes) Red rubber catheter/tubing.
*Advanced Reference:* Often used for digit (fingers/toes) tourniquet application.

**Jargon**   *Quick Reference:* Incoherent speech.
*Advanced Reference:* Can be referred to medical terminology that is not easily understood by the lay public.

**Jaundice**   *Quick Reference:* A yellowish discolourisation of the skin, whites of the eyes (conjunctiva) and mucous membrane.
*Advanced Reference:* Caused by deposition of the bile pigment, bilirubin, being present in the blood and tissues. Bile pigment accumulates in the blood if (i) too much is formed, (ii) the liver cells do not dispose of it, (iii) the bile ducts are obstructed. A trace of jaundice is common in the first few days of life but is not usually a serious matter.

**Jaw thrust**   *Quick Reference:* Procedure used for establishing a clear airway.
*Advanced Reference:* Involves lifting the patients jaw forward from its normal anatomical position therefore lifting the patients tongue from resting and causing obstruction of the oral cavity. Useful with patients who have cervical neck injury.

**Jejunosotomy**   *Quick Reference:* An artificial opening into the *jejunum*.
*Advanced Reference:* The insertion of a feeding catheter into the jejunum. It is performed when there is obstruction of the gastric system more superior to the jejunum or in gastric surgery cases where a partial gastrectomy may have been performed. The feeding tube gives a direct route for liquid nutrients to be inserted into the jejunum to follow the normal path of absorption.

**Jejunum**   *Quick Reference:* A section of small bowel directly after the duodenum.
*Advanced Reference:* The jejunum is approximately 2.4 m in length in the normal adult and supports the absorption and nutrients from the breakdown of food substance by gastric enzymes. Absorption of the nutrients is through the presence of villi in the lining of the jejunum and the continual movement of food substance by peristalsis. The jejunum connects to the ileum.

**Jelly**   *Quick Reference:* A term used to indicate lubricating jelly.

*Advanced Reference:* Often referred to during procedures where a level of lubrication is required, e.g. urology, gynaecology, general surgery, etc. However, *jelly* is commonly used in anaesthetic procedures for introducing an endotracheal (ET) tube with a bougie or stylette. It is also used in endoscopic procedures for insertion of scopes for diagnostic investigations. Generally speaking, this involves a water-based solution such as KY jelly; however, this is often mistaken for lignocaine jelly. Lignocaine jelly (2%) is used to localise sensitive areas for patients under local anaesthesia, which helps prevent discomfort during procedures such as flexible cystoscopy.

**Jelonet**   *Quick Reference:* Brand name for paraffin gauze.

*Advanced Reference:* Wound dressing impregnated with paraffin jelly used for burns and wounds.

**Jet ventilator**   *Quick Reference:* Type of high frequency patient ventilator.

*Advanced Reference:* The jet ventilator was designed to deliver very high respiratory rate frequencies i.e. 200/300 p.m. combined with small tidal volumes. Designed for use in ICU etc for patients with chest injuries or low compliance.

**Jewellers' forceps**   *Quick Reference:* Fine non-toothed dissecting forceps.

*Advanced Reference:* Jewellers forceps are used during microvascular surgery to dissect tissues or to hold the end of vessels or delicate tissue while operating under direct vision via a surgical microscope.

**Jewellery**   *Quick Reference:* With reference to theatre, controversy still exists regarding the wearing of jewellery by staff but in relation to patients the universal policy is still to either remove where possible or securely cover.

*Advanced Reference:* With regards to staff, in general it is accepted that jewellery should not be worn in theatre as it can harbour bacteria as well as being a danger by falling into wounds or scratching patients. However, the removal of wedding rings is optional as this can contravene human rights.

**Jobson Horn probe**   *Quick Reference:* Non-traumatic curette.

*Advanced Reference:* The probe has a small circular shape on the end of a fine shaft. The purpose of the probe is to scoop out any ear cavity content such as ear wax and foreign objects.

**Joint**   *Quick Reference:* The point where two or more bones meet.
*Advanced Reference:* An articulation.

**Jolls retractor**   *Quick Reference:* A retractor used during thyroid surgery.
*Advanced Reference:* Half-moon shaped with a spring-loaded towel clip on either end. The clamp is placed at each side of the surgical incision

at approximately right angles with each towel clip holding the skin edge. The middle knurled adjuster is used to expand the two ends of the clamp outwards creating maximum exposure of the surgical area.

**Joule**   *Quick Reference:* (jule) SI unit of energy.

*Advanced reference:* Joule refers to energy or amount of work done. Sometimes equated to watts per second. Most commonly encountered as the power source on defibrillators.

**J-pouch**   *Quick Reference:* Faecal reservoir.

*Advanced Reference:* Formed surgically by folding over the lower end of the ileum in an ileo-anal anastomosis.

**J-suture**   *Quick Reference:* J-shaped multi-use surgical suture needle.

*Advanced Reference:* The unique shape enables the surgeon to close deep layers of the wound without perforation of the underlying organs. Also used to close *laparoscopic* trocar incisions. Available in eyed and eyeless design allowing for choice of suture material.

**Judd Allis tissue forceps**   *Quick Reference:* Tissue forceps used to hold tissue without traumatising the structure.

*Advanced Reference:* Judd Allis have a slightly bevelled jaws that can be used to grip or hold delicate tissue without causing trauma.

**Jugular**   *Quick Reference:* Jugular vein situated on both lateral sides of the trachea.

*Advanced Reference:* There is an internal and external jugular vein commonly feeding into the superior vena cava returning deoxygenated blood to the right atrium of the heart. The external jugular is more visible because of its superficial position under the skin surface. It is regularly used for insertion of a central venous pressure (CVP) line and can be identified by using adjacent landmarks.

**Juxtaposition:**   *Quick Reference:* To position side by side.

*Advanced Reference:* The act of placing two or more things side by side or adjacent to one another.

**J-wire**   *Quick Reference:* Flexible wire with curved J-tip.

*Advanced Reference:* Used as an introduction aid for venous and arterial cannulation.

**Kaltostat**   *Quick Reference:* Type of wound dressing.

*Advanced Reference:* These dressings absorb exudate from wounds and turn to a gel which is then easily removed by syringing with saline. The gel also provides a moist covering for wound surfaces which enhances normal healing.

**Kaolin**   *Quick Reference:* (kao-lin) Compound used in the treatment of diarrhoea.

*Advanced Reference:* Sometimes mixed with morphine (kaolin–morph). Original source is China clay.

**Kefzol**   *Quick Reference:* Proprietary antibiotic.
*Advanced Reference:* A preparation of the cephalosporin, cephazolin.

**Kellers**   *Quick Reference:* An operation to correct deformity of the big toe.
*Advanced Reference:* Also referred to as *halux* **valgus** procedure. Commonly identified as a bunion.

**Keloid**   *Quick Reference:* (keel-oid) An overgrowth of scar tissue at the site of a wound.

*Advanced Reference:* Associated with scar tissue, instead of gradually disappearing the affected area spreads and causes puckering of the surrounding skin.

**Kelvin**   *Quick Reference:* SI unit of temperature.
*Advanced Reference:* Based on an absolute temperature scale where zero K is the temperature at which molecular motion ceases.

**Keratome**   *Quick Reference:* Surgical knife used in ophthalmic surgery.
*Advanced Reference:* A trowel-shaped blade for incising the cornea.

**Kerrison Rongeur**   *Quick Reference:* Bone nibbler.
*Advanced Reference:* Used in *orthopaedics* and neurosurgery, e.g. *laminectomy*. Available with an upward or downward bite.

**Ketamine**   *Quick Reference:* Anaesthetic agent. Alternative name is ketalar.
*Advanced Reference:* Termed a dissociative anaesthetic agent. May be given intravenously (IV) or intramuscularly (IM). Known to produce hallucinations and nightmares.

**Ketones**   *Quick Reference:* Products of incomplete fat metabolism.

*Advanced Reference:* Ketones are compounds containing the carboxyl group. Seen in relation to diabetic patients and acknowledged as being present by the breath having a smell resembling 'pear drops'. Poisoning by ketones is termed *ketosis*.

**Ketorolac**   *Quick Reference:* A non-steroidal anti-inflammatory drug (NSAID).

*Advanced Reference:* Has moderate analgesic affects combined with anti-inflammatory action.

**Key(ed) filling system**   *Quick Reference:* System for filling anaesthetic vaporisers.

*Advanced Reference:* Designed to prevent filling with an incorrect agent as well as preventing spillage and consequent pollution.

**Key hole surgery**   *Quick Reference:* Slang term for *minimally invasive surgical procedures*.

*Advanced Reference:* Indicates the use of telescopes as an alternative to open surgery.

**kHz**   *Quick Reference:* kilohertz.

*Advanced Reference:* The unit of frequency.

**Kidney**   *Quick Reference:* One of the two organs sited in the lumbar region.

*Advanced Reference:* Part of the urinary system and responsible for producing urine. Other functions include filtration of blood, maintenance of pH, re-absorption and secretion of salts and sugars, adjustment of blood pressure (BP), etc.

**Kidney bridge**   *Quick Reference:* Elevation facility incorporated into some operating tables.

*Advanced Reference:* The bridge is integral to the table design and is elevated during kidney surgery when the patient is in the lateral position. Intended to give better visualisation and access to the upper kidney area during surgery. Sometimes used in combination with jack-knifing of the table but improper use can lead to injury and reports of vena-caval occlusion have been reported.

**Kidney sling**   *Quick Reference:* A surgical sundry used to position and lower the kidney during transplantation.

*Advanced Reference:* Used by some surgeons during renal transplantation. The sling can prevent unnecessary handling of the kidney during surgery. Also to lower the kidney into the correct anatomical position prior to anastomosis of the *vein*, *artery* and then *ureter*.

**Kilogram**   *Quick Reference:* SI unit of mass.

*Advanced Reference:* Equal to 1000 grams. Kilo denotes a factor of 1000.

**Kinetics**   *Quick Reference:* Pertains to or indicates motion.
*Advanced Reference:* The science of the relations between the motion of bodies and the forces acting upon them.

**Kinnins**   *Quick Reference:* Substances present in the body and are powerful vasodilators.
*Advanced Reference:* Also thought to be involved in inducing pain and play a part in the production of allergy and anaphylaxis.

**Kiss of life**   *Quick Reference:* Also termed mouth-to-mouth or mouth-to-nose.
*Advanced Reference:* Relates to the expired air method of artificial respiration as used in cardiopulmonary resuscitation (CPR).

***Klebsiella***   *Quick Reference:* A type of bacteria.
*Advanced Reference:* Short bacilli, Gram-negative and non-spore-forming bacteria which can cause infection of the lung, intestines and urinary tract.

**Knee**   *Quick Reference:* The joint between the *femur* and *tibia*.
*Advanced Reference:* A hinge joint formed between the lower end of the femur and the upper end of the tibia.

**Knee elbow**   *Quick Reference:* Surgical operating position.
*Advanced Reference:* There are a number of variations to this position which is used mainly for spinal surgery. Involves the patient being placed in a crouched position, sometimes over a frame, with the patient resting on their knees and elbows. Due to the precarious nature of this position, there are many inherent and potential hazards. Also referred to as knee–chest position.

**Knife**   *Quick Reference:* Surgical scalpel.
*Advanced Reference:* Indicates both the handle and interchangeable blades used during surgery.

**Kochers forceps**   *Quick Reference:* (cock-ers) Toothed forceps.
*Advanced Reference:* A toothed self-retaining forceps used to hold or slippery tissues that require extra grip.

**Korotkoff (sounds)**   *Quick Reference:* Sounds heard when stethoscope is placed over the brachial artery.
*Advanced Reference:* The sounds are thought to be due to vibration caused by blood turbulence within the artery.

**Kraske's position**   *Quick Reference:* (kras-keys) Modification of the prone position.
*Advanced Reference:* Useful in proctological procedures for surgical access to the anal and rectal region. Variation of the *jack-knife* position.

**KUB**   *Quick Reference:* Abbreviation for kidney, ureter and bladder.
*Advanced Reference:* Used in radiographical examination to determine location, size, shape and malformation of the above organs.

**Kuntscher nail**   *Quick Reference:* An orthopaedic device used in fracture repair.

*Advanced Reference:* An *intramedullary* nail used for long bone fractures such as in the *femur*.

**Kyphosis**   *Quick Reference:* (kie-fosis) Curvature of the spine.

*Advanced Reference:* The curvature is directed in a concave manner directed forward giving a hunchback appearance.

**K (vitamin)**   *Quick Reference:* Fat-soluble vitamin group involved in blood coagulation.

*Advanced Reference:* Vitamin K is required for the formation of the enzyme thrombin, without which blood cannot clot. Formed in the body by intestinal bacteria, occurs in green vegetables and there are various synthetic versions. Can only be absorbed in the presence of bile, therefore if the flow of bile is obstructed vitamin K is poorly taken up. Newborn babies are sometimes short of vitamin K and so to prevent bleeding they are given the vitamin until bacteria in the intestine take over.

# L

**Labetalol**   *Quick Reference:* Drug used to treat hypertension.

*Advanced Reference:* It is a combined alpha- and beta-blocking drug. Used for the treatment of hypertension. In theatres, utilised as an infusion for lowering blood pressure (BP) in order to reduce blood loss. Drug used to treat hypertension. Available as Trandate.

**Labia**   *Quick Reference:* A lip.

*Advanced Reference:* There are two pairs of labia at the entrance to the *vagina*, the *labia majora* and *labia minora* which together form part of the female external genitalia known as the *vulva*.

**Labile**   *Quick Reference:* Indicates something prone to frequent swings and changes; unstable.

*Advanced Reference:* Term frequently applied to a patient's BP that is prone to frequent swings and changes.

**Labour**   *Quick Reference:* The process of giving birth (parturition).

*Advanced Reference:* Labour consists of three stages: *first stage* starts with the onset of labour pains, etc. until there is full dilatation of the cervical os; *second stage* lasts until the baby is delivered; *third stage*, continues until the placenta is expelled.

**Labyrinth**   *Quick Reference:* (lab-rinth) Any intricate or involved enclosure.

*Advanced Reference:* The labyrinth of the ear consists of the cochlea and semicircular canals which form the inner ear and are the organs of balance and hearing. The *bony labyrinth* indicates the bony canals of the inner ear and the *membranous labyrinth* is the soft structure inside the bony canals. Labyrinthectomy is excision of the labyrinth and labyrintitis (which causes vertigo, is inflammation of the labyrinth).

**Laceration**   *Quick Reference:* (lass-air-ashun) The act of tearing.

*Advanced Reference:* A laceration is a wound with torn and ragged edges, as opposed to an incision or cut.

**Lacri-lube**   *Quick Reference:* Form of liquid paraffin used as an eye lubricant.

*Advanced Reference:* Used to protect and lubricate the eyes and assist in keeping them closed during anaesthesia.

L

**Lacrimal**   *Quick Reference:* Pertaining to tears.
*Advanced Reference:* Refers to the parts or structures concerned with the secretion and drainage of tears. Lacrimation is the act of shedding tears, crying.

**Lactase**   *Quick Reference:* An enzyme of the intestinal juice.
*Advanced Reference:* Lactase is involved in the breakdown of *lactose* into dextrose and galactose.

**Lactation**   *Quick Reference:* Formation of milk.
*Advanced Reference:* Commonly refers to breast milk and the period during which the child is nourished from the breast.

**Lacteals**   *Quick Reference:* Lymphatic capillary or duct. Having the consistency of milk.
*Advanced Reference:* Lymphatic ducts in the small intestine which absorb digested fats.

**Lactic acid**   *Quick Reference:* It is an end product of *glucose* metabolism.
*Advanced Reference*: A compound produced in muscles by the breakdown of glucose in the absence of oxygen. Formed when there is an oxygen debt in exercise and responsible for muscle cramp.

**Lactose**   *Quick Reference:* Milk sugar.
*Advanced Reference:* A compound of the simple sugars, galactose and glucose. In the intestine the galactose is broken down to form glucose.

**Lahey swab**   *Quick Reference:* (lay-he) Small swab used for blunt dissection. Also known as a pledget and peanut.
*Advanced Reference:* Used in many surgical specialities especially vascular and are always used mounted on an instrument such as an artery forcep. Although referred to as a swab, its main intention is for blunt dissection rather than absorption of blood.

**Laminar**   *Quick Reference:* Laminar flow refers to a type of air flow system utilised in operating theatres.
*Advanced Reference:* An air flow system used mainly in orthopaedic theatres to remove particulate matter and *fungi* from the air and so aiding the prevention of airborne infections during open surgical procedures. The flow is in one direction only and at high velocity.

**Laminectomy**   *Quick Reference:* General term applied to spinal surgery.
*Advanced Reference:* The name indicates removal of the lamina and is a procedure for treating a number of spinal-related problems, i.e. tumours, prolapsed disc, relieve pressure, etc.

**Lancet**   *Quick Reference:* Surgical knife.
*Advanced Reference:* It is of a two-edged pointed design and originally used for opening abscesses and blood letting.

**Landmarks**   *Quick Reference:* Refers to anatomical landmarks used in anaesthesia and surgery.

*Advanced Reference:* Most commonly used are ileac crest, umbilicus, xyphoid process and sternal notch.

**Langenbeck**   *Quick Reference:* Name of a number of different surgical instruments.

*Advanced Reference:* More usually a retractor but there is also a Langenbeck periosteal elevator.

**Langer's lines**   *Quick Reference:* Anatomical lines along which most of the supporting fibres in the skin are arranged.

*Advanced Reference:* They determine the direction in which the skin folds if pinched. Are of concern in surgery in that incisions along them are less likely to stretch than those at a diagonal to them, therefore affecting the cosmetic outcome.

**Lanolin**   *Quick Reference:* Fat obtained from sheep's wool.

*Advanced Reference:* Used as a base for ointments, one reason being that it can penetrate the skin. It is capable of absorbing and mixing with water but can cause sensitisation and provoke a reaction.

**Laparoscopic**   *Quick Reference:* The term used to imply insertion of a scope into the abdominal cavity.

*Advanced Reference:* This approach can be used to remove colon, gallbladder, spleen, uterus or even tubal ligation (female sterilisation).

**Laparoscopy**   *Quick Reference:* Endoscopic examination of a body (abdominal) cavity using a laparoscope.

*Advanced Reference:* The **endoscope** is introduced through the abdominal wall into the peritoneum following insufflation of **carbon dioxide** to create a **pneumoperitoneum**. This enhanced space then improves vision and access.

**Laparotomy**   *Quick Reference:* Surgical opening of the abdominal cavity.

*Advanced Reference:* Used commonly to indicate a surgical exploration of the abdomen.

**Largactil**   *Quick Reference:* Drug used primarily as a tranquilliser.

*Advanced Reference:* A preparation of chlorpromazine hydrochloride and also used as an antipsychotic.

**Large intestine**   *Quick Reference:* The bowel.

*Advanced Reference:* It is approximately 1.5 m long, sits draped around the **small intestine** and consists of the caecum, ascending colon, transverse colon, descending colon, sigmoid colon, rectum and anal canal.

**Laryngeal mask airway**   *Quick Reference:* LMA.

*Advanced Reference:* Invented in 1983, sometimes described as a midway option between an oro/nasopharyngeal airway and an endotracheal (ET) tube. Designed to provide a patient airway without the need for laryngoscopy as it lies above the vocal cords rather than below them and so not requiring muscle-relaxing drugs. It is said to have replaced upwards of 40% of intubations in the theatre setting. There are now a number of variations available but currently the original LMA remains the most popular. Following on from the original design, there is now a full paediatric range, flexible model and more recently the intubating version.

**Laryngectomy**   *Quick Reference:* (lar-in-jec-tommy) Removal of the *larynx*.

*Advanced Reference:* Removal of part or all of the larynx usually to treat advanced stages of cancer.

**Laryngoscope**   *Quick Reference:* (lar-in-gos-copy) An instrument for looking into or examining the larynx.

*Advanced Reference:* An illuminated device of varying design primarily used in anaesthesia for insertion of an ET tube.

**Laryngospasm**   *Quick Reference:* Spasmodic closure of the larynx.

*Advanced Reference:* Involves closure or partial closure of the vocal cords and so obscuring the entrance to the larynx/trachea and starving the patient of oxygen. Many causes but common at induction of anaesthesia and extubation due to irritation of the vocal cords by secretions, suction catheter, etc. Treatment can involve administration of *suxamethonium* to bring about relaxation of the cords and so allow intubation if necessary and oxygenation.

**Larynx**   *Quick Reference:* (lar-inks) Voice box. Visible lump at the front of the neck which is the thyroid cartilage of the larynx (**Adam's apple**).

*Advanced Reference:* The chief function of the larynx is the production of the voice, as it contains the *vocal cords*. It is lined with mucous membrane continuous with the throat above and trachea below.

**Laser**   *Quick Reference:* Light amplification by stimulated emission of radiation.

*Advanced Reference:* Laser is the application of the fact that light is a form of energy. In *ordinary light* the energy is diffused but with a *laser* the beam is concentrated and organised. Utilised as a cutting and coagulating aid in numerous types of surgeries.

**Lasix**   *Quick Reference:* Proprietary diuretic drug.

*Advanced Reference:* Alternatively known as frusemide. A loop diuretic used in heart failure, kidney failure and general oedema. Works by inhibiting reabsorption in the Loop of Henle.

**Latent heat**   *Quick Reference:* Heat which is used to bring about a change in state, not in temperature.

*Advanced Reference:* Refers to the energy requirement in order to change the state of any substance and in the process, does not create a temperature change as in a liquid to a gas, solid to a liquid, etc.

**Lateral**   *Quick Reference:* Indicates to the side.

*Advanced Reference:* Away from the midline. In surgery, left lateral indicates the patient lying on their left side.

**Latex**   *Quick Reference:* Latex rubber. Initially a milky fluid of the rubber plant made up of various gums, resins, fats and waxes.

*Advanced Reference:* The source of rubber and is used in numerous hospital-based products with surgical gloves being one of the more familiar.

**Latex agglutination test**   *Quick Reference:* Carried out to detect the presence of the rheumatoid factor.

*Advanced Reference:* A test carried out in the diagnosis of rheumatoid arthritis.

**Latex allergy**   *Quick Reference:* Hypersensitivity to latex.

*Advanced Reference:* Allergic reaction most commonly connected with the wearing of latex gloves in theatres, correctly called *contact dermatitis*. Reactions can range from minor redness to full *anaphylactic* reaction. Due to proteins in the latex (but originally there was indecision over the primary source), with glove powder, starches and various chemicals used in their manufacture being suspected. There are alternatives for scrub staff and wherever possible non-scrubbed staff can be supplied with a number of polyvinyl chloride (PVC)-related products.

**Latissimus dorsi**   *Quick Reference:* Muscle of the back region.

*Advanced Reference:* It is the flat back muscle which covers the central and lower back. Said to be the largest muscle in the body.

**Laughing gas**   *Quick Reference:* Nitrous oxide.

*Advanced Reference:* Anecdotally said to produce euphoria and a feeling of happiness. Nitrous oxide has both anaesthetic and analgesic properties.

**Lavage**   *Quick Reference:* (lav-arge) To wash out (a cavity).

*Advanced Reference:* Indicates to wash out a body cavity, e.g. *peritoneal lavage, pulmonary lavage*.

**Lead apron**   *Quick Reference:* Radiation protection device.

*Advanced Reference:* Worn during surgical procedures when X-ray is being used. Fits over the shoulders and should be of adequate length to cover the reproductive organs. Comprised of a lead interior covered with plastic or leather. Great care should be taken in handling and storage as the lead interior is prone to cracking, and so lose the protective properties.

**LeFort**   *Quick Reference:* A classification of facial fractures.

*Advanced Reference:* The LeFort classification is a useful tool to determine the appropriate method of reduction and stabilisation. LeFort 1 is a transverse fracture of the maxilla. LeFort 2 is a pyramidal fracture of the frontal process of the maxilla, the nasal bones and the orbital floor. LeFort 3 includes both zygomas, namely maxillas and nasal bones; also the ethmoid, sphenoid and outer orbital bones.

**Legionnaire's disease**   *Quick Reference:* Disease spread via airborne water droplets.

*Advanced Reference:* The name stems from an outbreak of a pneumonia-like disease which occurred in Philadelphia in 1976 at a convention of the American Legion in which 29 people died. As a result, a new organism was identified and named *Legionella pneumophilia*. Cannot be spread from person to person. Common cause, as with the original outbreak, is water-cooled, air-conditioning systems that have not been regularly maintained. This commonly involves the addition of chlorine to the water reservoir.

**Lens**   *Quick Reference:* A biconvex structure behind the iris involved in focusing of the eye.

*Advanced Reference:* A flexible structure, the size of a lentil which adjusts the focus as the surrounding muscle increases or decreases its curvature.

**Lesion**   *Quick Reference:* Non-specific term referring to the damage done to tissues.

*Advanced Reference:* Involves a pathological change in a body tissue. Any change or damage may be due to injury or a disease process.

**Lesser curvature**   *Quick Reference:* Concave curve of the stomach.

*Advanced Reference:* It is the boundary of the stomach that forms a short concave curvature on the right side between the oesophagus and duodenum.

**Lethidrone**   *Quick Reference:* Alternative name is *nalorphine*. A narcotic antagonist.

*Advanced Reference:* Nalorphine neutralises the action of morphine, pethidine and drugs with similar actions.

**Leuc(o)-**   *Quick Reference:* Prefix indicating white.

*Advanced Reference:* Used in relation to both white cells and white matter in the brain.

**Leucocyte**   *Quick Reference:* The white cells in the blood.

*Advanced Reference:* The total number is raised in infection while being abnormally low in other conditions. *Leucocytosis* indicates an increase in white cell count and *leucopaenia*, a decrease.

**Leucotomy**   *Quick Reference:* Operation on the brain.
   *Advanced Reference:* Involves cutting certain fibres (frontothalmic) in the brain as a treatment of some insanity disorders. The original operation involved injecting alcohol to destroy the fibres.

**Leukaemia**   *Quick Reference:* Malignant disease involving overproduction of white blood cells.
   *Advanced Reference:* May be acute or chronic and according to the type involved can be divided into myeloid or lymphatic.

**Levobupivacaine**   *Quick Reference:* Local anaesthetic (LA) drug.
   *Advanced Reference:* Very similar in action to **bupivacaine** but requires a much larger dose to produce the same effects.

**Levophed**   *Quick Reference:* A vasoconstrictor drug.
   *Advanced Reference:* It is in fact a noradrenaline and used to raise the BP in severe hypotension and/or cardiac arrest.

**LFA**   *Quick Reference:* Low-friction arthroplasty.
   *Advanced Reference:* Refers to the Charnley (Sir John) total hip replacement. Made of stainless steel with a small femoral head, high-density **polyethylene** cup and secured with acrylic **cement**.

**Ligaclip**   *Quick Reference:* A metallic surgical clip used for haemostasis.
   *Advanced Reference:* The ligaclip is applied on a ligaclip applicator. Ligaclips are placed on a vessel and pinched shut; the clips occlude the lumen and stop the vessels from bleeding.

**Ligament**   *Quick Reference:* Fibrous band between two bones at a joint.
   *Advanced Reference:* Ligaments are flexible but inelastic. They come into play only at the extremes of movement and cannot be stretched when they are taut.

**Ligature**   *Quick Reference:* Material used for sewing or tying. *Ligation* is to tie.
   *Advanced Reference:* Generally involves body tissues and vessels, and can be of synthetic or natural origin, e.g. nylon, silk, wire, catgut as well as patients own tendon, fascia, etc.

**Lignocaine**   *Quick Reference:* A local anaesthetic (LA) drug.
   *Advanced Reference:* Also termed *lidocaine*. Used in various percentage strengths and sometimes with adrenaline added to act as a vasoconstrictor. Also used as an anti-arrhythmic agent in the management of ventricular tachycardia and ventricular *ectopic* beats. Ointment and gel versions, usually 2% are available for use on e.g. urethra. Also available as a 4% throat spray.

**Limbus**   *Quick Reference:* A border or edge of certain structures.
   *Advanced Reference:* The limbus of the eye is where the cornea joins the conjunctiva.

L

**Linctus**   *Quick Reference:* A syrup.
*Advanced Reference:* Medium used to carry medicines, i.e. cough mixtures.

**Linea alba**   *Quick Reference:* A fibrous band.
*Advanced Reference:* A fibrous band running vertically along the entire length of the anterior abdominal wall and receives the attachments of the oblique and tranversalis muscles of the abdomen.

**Linear**   *Quick Reference:* Of length. Indicating one dimension.
*Advanced Reference:* Indicates one direction in a straight path. When particles travel in a straight line and not in closed orbits. X-rays travel in straight lines prior to a degree of scatter. In *laminar* flow systems the air travels in a linear manner, i.e. straight lines.

**Linen**   *Quick Reference:* Term used to generally indicate theatre clothing, etc.
*Advanced Reference:* All theatre-related clothing, drapes, instrument wrapping, etc. are included within this term, even though today many are made from synthetic materials.

**Lingual**   *Quick Reference:* Of the tongue.
*Advanced Reference:* Term used to indicate the tongue.

**Lipaemia**   *Quick Reference:* (lip-eem-ea) Excess fat in the blood.
*Advanced Reference:* Often associated with diabetes. Can also include *cholesterol*.

**Lipase**   *Quick Reference:* An enzyme.
*Advanced Reference:* Lipase is involved in the breaking down of fats and is present in pancreatic juice and assists in converting them to fatty acids and glycerol.

**Lipid**   *Quick Reference:* Fatty substance.
*Advanced Reference:* A group of fatty substances that are insoluble in water but soluble in alcohol, and form an important part of the diet.

**Lip(o)-**   *Quick Reference:* Prefix for fat.
*Advanced Reference:* Lipid, lipoid refer to fat-like substances such as *cholesterol*.

**Lipoma**   *Quick Reference:* **Benign** tumour often occurring just below the skin.
*Advanced Reference:* Lipomas are harmless and composed of fat cells.

**Liposuction**   *Quick Reference:* Surgical removal of fat-utilising suction.
*Advanced Reference:* The surgical removal of fat deposits, especially for cosmetic reasons. The suction device is usually inserted endoscopically. Also known as suction lipectomy.

**Lithium**   *Quick Reference:* Metallic element.

*Advanced Reference:* It is used in the treatment of manic depression. More recently has been used in ointment form as a treatment for types of dermatitis.

**Lithopaxy**   *Quick Reference:* Crushing of a bladder stone.
*Advanced Reference:* Carried out with a lithotrite, followed by irrigation to flush out the crushed fragments.

**Lithotomy**   *Quick Reference:* Originally used to indicate cutting into the bladder to remove a stone. The patient for this was positioned with legs elevated into various designs of *stirrups*, i.e. legs raised and slightly head down, hence the position became known as *lithotomy*.
*Advanced Reference:* The lithotomy position is when the patient is supine with their legs up in stirrups. This is often used in **gynaecology** or **urology**. Placing the legs in this position must be carried out in synchronus, in order to avoid injury to the spinal column and associated structures.

**Lithotomy tray**   *Quick Reference:* Instrument tray used when the patient is in the lithotomy position.
*Advanced Reference:* A table attachment which fits into the operating table when the end section has been removed. Used commonly in gynaecology for holding instruments.

**Lithotripsy**   *Quick Reference:* The crushing of a stone.
*Advanced Reference:* Procedure for breaking down renal stones, either directly or using shock waves (extracorporeal shock wave lithotripsy, ESWL).

**Lithotrite**   *Quick Reference:* Urological instrument.
*Advanced Reference:* Instrument used to crush urinary bladder stones.

**Litmus**   *Quick Reference:* Naturally occurring blue colouring matter.
*Advanced Reference:* Litmus is turned red by acids and restored to blue by an alkali.

**Liver**   *Quick Reference:* Literal meaning is *gland.* Hepatic indicates the liver.
*Advanced Reference:* The largest gland in the human body situated in the right upper area of the abdominal cavity, just below the diaphragm. Performs many functions, i.e. secretes bile; removes toxins from the blood; removes nitrogen from amino acids; stores vitamins A, B12, D, E and K; stores iron and glycogen; produces heat and converts stored fat into other fatty products (cholesterol), glycogen to glucose when needed and metabolises proteins.

**Live-related donor**   *Quick Reference:* Term used with reference to *transplantation*.
*Advanced Reference:* The term is used mainly in renal transplantation and refers to a donor kidney being from a live relative rather than the alternative donor method, **cadaver**.

**Lloyd-Davies stirrups**   *Quick Reference:* Type of lithotomy poles.
*Advanced Reference:* More versatile type of lithotomy stirrup that has a number of adjustable joints and anatomically shaped lower leg rests into which the patients calves can be secured. They allow for variations in positioning and are designed for use with longer operations.

**Lobe**   *Quick Reference:* A well-defined part of an organ.
*Advanced Reference:* Partitions of tissue as found in the lungs, thyroid, etc. *Lobectomy* is the removal of only the lobe and not the entire organ itself.

**Lobotomy**   *Quick Reference:* Neurosurgery procedure.
*Advanced Reference:* An operation on the prefrontal area of the brain designed to bring about behavioural change through severing nerve fibres.

**Local anaesthetic**   *Quick reference:* LA. Involves anaesthetising (localising) one specific area of the body.
*Advanced Reference:* Also termed regional anaesthesia. Can involve infiltration, surface creams as well as epidural and spinal techniques using various forms of LA agents.

**Locomotor**   *Quick Reference:* Relating to movement.
*Advanced Reference:* Usually refers to human movement and involves nerves and muscles as well as bones and joints.

**Log-roll**   *Quick Reference:* System used for turning injured patients.
*Advanced Reference:* Used when a patient has suspected or confirmed spinal injury. Involves rolling the patient as a unit, with no twisting of the spine and trunk. Requires a minimum of four to six people for the technique to be carried out satisfactorily. Some variations, such as first-aid settings, involve tying the patient's legs together and securing the arms to the sides of the body as additional stabilisation.

**Loin**   *Quick Reference:* Area of the back immediately above the buttocks.
*Advanced Reference:* The area that extends between the **thorax** (lower ribs) and the **pelvis (iliac crest)**.

**Lomodex**   *Quick Reference:* Proprietary form of **dextran**.
*Advanced Reference:* A plasma substitute used in infusion with either saline or glucose to increase volume. Also used to prevent thrombosis following surgery. Available in two strengths: 40 and 70.

**Lomotil**   *Quick Reference:* Medicinal preparation used in treatment of diarrhoea.
*Advanced Reference:* It is a mixture of diphenoxylate hydrochloride and atropine. It reduces gut motility and allows time for water absorption from the faeces.

**Lorazepam**   *Quick Reference:* Antidepressant and anxiolytic.
*Advanced Reference:* One of the benzodiazepines used to treat anxiety, insomnia and as a pre-med. Available as Ativan.

**Lordosis**   *Quick Reference:* Curvature of the spine.

*Advanced Reference:* Indicates towards the front. As with the natural curvature in the *lumbar* region which produces the hollow of the back. *Kyphosis* is the opposite to lordosis.

**Lotion**   *Quick Reference:* Solutions or suspensions in water.

*Advanced Reference:* Lotions are used to carry medications as with skin treatments. Usually involves the drug being left behind after evaporation. Alcohol is usually added to assist the action. Common term for many skin preparations, often containing *hibitane*.

**Lubricant**   *Quick Reference:* Generally refers to substances used to make bodily entrance easier and less traumatic.

*Advanced Reference:* KY jelly is a universally used lubricant, easy to use and water soluble. There are also lubricants containing LAs usually in a 2% strength of lignocaine and hibitane cream used mainly in obstetrics to lubricate the vulva during labour and childbirth. Besides being used on fingers, etc. for examination, are coated on instruments such as rigid scopes to facilitate easier passage.

**Lucid**   *Quick Reference:* Relates to a clear state of the mind.

*Advanced Reference:* Indicates clear logical thinking.

**Luer**   *Quick Reference:* Connecting system for cannulae, etc.

*Advanced Reference:* Originally just one of a number of connecting systems for intravenous (IV) sets, cannulae, etc. Now universally used and adapted to a 'Luer-Lock' system.

**Lumbar**   *Quick Reference:* The part of the back between the lowest pair of ribs and the top of the *pelvis*.

*Advanced Reference:* The lumbar region is supported by the five lumbar *vertebrae*. The lumbar plexus is a group of nerves that supplies the skin and muscles of the lower abdomen, thighs and groin.

**Lumbar puncture**   *Quick Reference:* Access into the spinal canal.

*Advanced Reference:* Involves the introduction of a needle into the spinal canal in order to draw off a specimen of cerebrospinal fluid (CSF) for examination.

**Lumen**   *Quick Reference:* Space inside a tube.

*Advanced Reference:* Indicates the cavity or space inside a tubular structure, as with the lumen of a blood vessel.

**Lungs**   *Quick Reference:* Main organs of respiration.

*Advanced Reference:* The lungs allow the exchange of gases into and out of the blood. Positioned either side of the heart/mediastinum with the left lung having two lobes and the right lung three. The lungs themselves are made up of alveoli, bronchioles, blood vessels, nerves, connective and elastic tissue.

**Lux**   *Quick Reference:* The unit of illumination.
*Advanced Reference:* Equivalent to one lumen per square metre of surface when measured at right angles to the direction of the light.

**Lymphatic**   *Quick Reference:* (lim-fat-ic) Referring to lymph.
*Advanced Reference:* Also the lymphatic system and circulation.

**Lymphocyte**   *Quick Reference:* (lim-fo-site) White blood cells concerned mainly with the immune system.
*Advanced Reference:* Lymphocytes are formed in the *lymph nodes* as well as in the *reticulo-endothelial* system. They are divided into two classes: B- and T-cells, the latter being formed in the *thymus* gland. B-cells produce antibodies.

**Lymphoma**   *Quick reference:* (lim-foam-a) Condition of the lymph glands.
*Advanced Reference:* Can be caused by *malignant* disease or *Hodgkin's disease*. Diagnosis usually made by lymph node biopsy and treated with *radiotherapy* or *chemotherapy*.

**Lysol**   *Quick Reference:* (lie-sol) A soapy solution once used as a household disinfectant.
*Advanced Reference:* It is caustic and highly irritant, hence its withdrawal from general use.

# M

**MAC** *Quick Reference:* Minimal alveolar concentration.

*Advanced Reference:* Refers to inhalational/volatile anaesthetic agents and is the minimum concentration of the agent in the alveoli that prevents a response to a surgical stimulus in 50% of subjects. Therefore, it is a measure of potency or the strength of the agent. MAC can be used to compare potencies of different agents, i.e. an agent with a low MAC value will require a lesser concentration than one with a high MAC value.

**Macintosh blade** *Quick Reference:* A curved laryngoscope blade used for intubation.

*Advanced Reference:* Refers to a curved adult laryngoscope blade designed to pass into the *vallecula* and lift local structures in order to facilitate intubation.

**Macrodex** *Quick Reference:* Proprietary form of Dextran 70.

*Advanced Reference:* Used intravenously (IV) as a plasma expander and to help prevent deep vein thrombosis (*DVT*). Available in *dextrose* or *saline* base.

**Macula** *Quick Reference:* Central area found in the *retina* containing the Fovea.

*Advanced Reference:* Central area of the retina, where vision is the clearest.

**Magill's forceps** *Quick Reference:* Angled forceps for introducing *endotracheal* (ET) tubes.

*Advanced Reference:* Ergonomically designed forceps used for grasping the ET tube as an aid to placement into the *larynx* and retrieving foreign bodies from the pharynx.

**Magnesium** *Quick Reference:* Metallic element.

*Advanced Reference:* Used as an antacid and in treatment of refractory ventricular fibrillation (VF).

**Malignant** *Quick Reference:* Term used to distinguish severe or progressive forms of a disease.

*Advanced Reference:* When used in relation to a tumour indicates cancerous as opposed to benign which is a simple growth that does not invade other tissues.

**Malleable**   *Quick Reference:* Pliable, able to be formed into a different shape.

*Advanced Reference:* Substance that is able to be re-shaped without tendency to return to original form. In relation to theatres as with anaesthetic *face masks*, intubating *stylette*, wound retractor, etc.

**Malpractice**   *Quick Reference:* Professional negligence.

*Advanced Reference:* Involves failure to exercise reasonable care and judgement which may result in injury or harm due to lack of professional knowledge, experience or skill, that can be expected of others in the same profession.

**Mandible**   *Quick Reference:* Lower jaw.

*Advanced Reference:* It is a single bone that is loosely jointed with the skull at the temporo-mandibular joint in front of the ear.

**Mannitol**   *Quick Reference:* A powerful *diuretic. Hypertonic solution.*

*Advanced Reference:* It is a form of carbohydrate. Therapeutically it is used to treat *oedema* and to decrease pressure in certain body areas, i.e. intracranial, eyeball in *glaucoma*, etc. Sometimes used to assist renal perfusion prior to clamping of the aorta during vascular surgery.

**Manometer**   *Quick Reference:* Device used for measuring pressure.

*Advanced Reference:* The manometer measures pressure by the use of a head of fluid moving against a measuring scale. Common example is with central venous pressure (CVP) measurement, where a column of fluid (saline) indicates pressure on a centimetres scale ($cmH_2O$).

**Manubrium**   *Quick Reference:* Or manubria. Upper section of the breastbone (sternum).

*Advanced Reference:* It articulates with the clavicle and the first costal cartilage.

**Marrow**   *Quick Reference:* Soft core of a bone.

*Advanced Reference:* At birth the bones are filled with red marrow but in adult life the red marrow of the limbs is replaced by yellow marrow consisting mainly of fat, however, in the rest of the skeleton red marrow persists. Red marrow is actively engaged in producing various blood cells.

**Marsupialisation**   *Quick Reference:* (mar-soup-eal-ise-ashun) To shell out, as from a pouch.

*Advanced Reference:* Example is marsupialisation of a cyst or abscess of the Bartholins gland of the vagina.

**Massive transfusion** *Quick Reference:* Definition involving blood replacement.

*Advanced Reference:* Although used as a term, is in fact a definition; Massive transfusion is replacement of half the patient's blood volume within one hour.

**Mastectomy** *Quick Reference:* Surgical removal of the breast.

*Advanced Reference:* Carried out in different forms. *Simple* is the removal of the breast alone whereas *radical* indicates removal of the breast, muscles and lymph nodes. *Lumpectomy* involves removal of a smaller lump or growth.

**Masticate** *Quick Reference:* To chew food.

*Advanced Reference:* Involves upper and lower jaws. Mastication breaks up food and mixes it with *saliva* which aids swallowing.

**Mastoid** *Quick Reference:* Bone situated behind the ear.

*Advanced Reference:* A knob of bone projecting down from the skull behind the ear and attaches to the front part of the *sternomastoid* muscle.

**Mastoidectomy** *Quick Reference:* Surgical removal of diseased bone.

*Advanced Reference:* Surgical removal of the diseased bone and drainage of the infected mastoid air cells.

**MAST suit** *Quick Reference:* Device used for initial resuscitation and transport. Military anti-shock trouser (MAST).

*Advanced Reference:* Theatre staff may encounter this during accident and emergency (A&E) resuscitation events. The principle involved is that the suit, once on the patient, can be inflated and by applying pressure reduces venous pooling and therefore aid the transfer of blood to central areas of greater need.

**Maxilla** *Quick Reference:* Jaw bone.

*Advanced Reference:* In particular, indicates the upper jaw.

**McCoy** *Quick Reference:* Laryngoscope blade.

*Advanced Reference:* The McCoy has a hinged tip which can be lifted up by pressing a lever connected to the handle of the laryngoscope. Can be used to lift up the *epiglottis* and improve the view of the *larynx*. Useful as an alternative to other blades (*Macintosh*) during difficult intubation situations.

**Mean** *Quick Reference:* Occupying a position midway between the extremes of a set of values.

*Advanced Reference:* Mean arterial pressure (MAP) is calculated by adding the systolic reading to two times the diastolic then dividing by three.

**Meatus**  *Quick Reference:* An opening or tunnel.
*Advanced Reference:* Present in many parts of the body, i.e. the ear (external acoustic meatus).

**Mecklel's diverticulum**  *Quick Reference:* A protrusion from the small intestine.
*Advanced Reference:* Said to be a vestigal structure representing the yolk stalk. Resembles the appendix and can become inflamed with symptoms like those of appendicitis.

**Meconium**  *Quick Reference:* Greenish fluid composed of bile and mucus present in an infants intestine.
*Advanced Reference:*It is passed soon after birth or prior to delivery, if labour is difficult.

**Median**  *Quick Reference:* In the middle.
*Advanced Reference:* The median plane divides the body into the left and right halves whereas medial indicates being towards the mid line.

**Mediastinum**  *Quick Reference:* Space in the middle of the thorax.
*Advanced Reference:* A compartment between the lungs containing the heart, major blood vessels, trachea and oesophagus.

**Medical air**  *Quick Reference:* Also known as compressed air.
*Advanced Reference:* Can be piped directly into theatres or in cylinders with a colour coding of grey body with white and black shoulder. Used mainly to drive pneumatic drills, etc. and some patient ventilators. Usually used at a pressure of 4 or 7 bar depending on equipment type.

**Medic-Alert**  *Quick Reference:* Refers to a database of patients suffering certain conditions and taking medication.
*Advanced Reference:* Members wear a bracelet or necklace indicating condition, etc. and contact details for detailed information.

**Medical Devices Agency**  *Quick Reference:* Body responsible for overseeing the safety and quality of all medical-related equipments used in UK hospitals.
*Advanced Reference:* The agency relies on liaison with all health care staff as well as manufacturers for information and feedback on safety and quality.

**Medical engineering**  *Quick Reference:* Refers to the department responsible for maintenance of hospital equipment.
*Advanced Reference:* Also referred to in some centres as the electrical biomedical engineering (EBME) department. Besides maintenance

responsibilities, these departments are also involved in purchasing and loaning of equipment.

**Medico-legal**  *Quick Reference:* Refers to the branch of law relating to medical aspects.

*Advanced Reference:* Medical negligence claims in the UK are rising annually and with it, medico-legal law has become a legal subspeciality in itself. At one time almost solely related to doctors but with changing emphasis on overall care and accountability; it now includes and involves all staff disciplines.

**Medrone**  *Quick Reference:* Proprietary preparation of the corticosteroid methylprednisolone.

*Advanced Reference:* Used as an anti-inflammatory mainly for *arthritis*, joint pain and allergies.

**Medulla**  *Quick Reference:* Innermost part of an organ or gland.

*Advanced Reference:* Examples are the *kidney* and *adrenal glands*. Also used to mean the *marrow* of a bone and spinal cord, and the *medulla oblongata* in the hindbrain region. In orthopaedic surgery, an intramedullary nail is one which is inserted lengthwise into the shaft of a bone to stabilise a fracture.

**Medulla oblongata**  *Quick Reference:* (medula-oblongarta) The lowest part of the brain. The portion of the spinal cord positioned inside the skull.

*Advanced Reference:* It contains the centres which govern the reflexes for breathing, heart rate and blood pressure.

**Mefoxin**  *Quick Reference:* Broad-spectrum antibiotic.

*Advanced Reference:* Produced in powder form for reconstitution. It is a preparation of the cephalosporin, cefoxitin.

**Mega**  *Quick Reference:* Huge, great. Also megalo, mego.

*Advanced Reference:* A quantity of one million times a given unit.

**Megacolon**  *Quick Reference:* Abnormal enlargement of the bowel.

*Advanced Reference:* Condition which may arise due to a number of causes one being *hirschsprungs disease.*

**Membrane**  *Quick Reference:* Thin layer of tissue composed of epithelial cells and connective tissue.

*Advanced Reference:* Covers surfaces, lines a cavity or divides a space within the body. Examples are mucous, serous, synovial.

**Mendelsons syndrome**  *Quick Reference:* Also termed aspiration pneumonitis or acid aspiration syndrome.

*Advanced Reference:* Inflammatory reaction following aspiration of gastric contents. First described in 1946 by a New York obstetrician when he discovered an asthma-like syndrome associated with a mottled appearance on X-ray. He considered this due to gastric acid contents with a pH of less than 2.5 entering the lungs. Can happen during induction and recovery from anaesthesia and more commonly with certain risk groups such as emergency surgery, *Caesarean section*, *hiatus hernia*, etc.

**Meniscus**  *Quick Reference:* Piece of cartilage separating joint surfaces.
*Advanced Reference:* Usually a semicircular or crescent-shaped section of cartilage, as in the knee joint.

**Menorrhagia**  *Quick Reference: (menor-ag-ea)* Excessive blood loss at the monthly period (*menstruation*).
*Advanced Reference:* Can be due to a number of factors including hormonal imbalance, clotting disorders and irregular ovulation.

**Menstruation**  *Quick Reference:* Female monthly period.
*Advanced Reference:* Involves the monthly loss of blood and mucous membrane (*endometrium*) lining the uterus following the expectation of pregnancy which has not occurred.

**Mesentery**  *Quick Reference:* A double layer of peritoneum which attaches the intestine to the posterior abdominal wall.
*Advanced Reference:* Carried within the mesentery are the blood and lymphatic vessels and nerves that supply the gut.

**Mesothelioma**  *Quick Reference:* A tumour of the pleura, peritoneum or pericardium.
*Advanced Reference:* Pleural mesothelioma; it is often due to *asbestos* exposure.

**Metabolism**  *Quick Reference:* Chemical process by which the substance of the body is produced and maintained.
*Advanced Reference:* Metabolism consists of *catabolism* (breakdown of molecules) and *anabolism* ( reconstruction of molecules).

**Metacarpal(s)**  *Quick Reference:* Bones of the hand/wrist.
*Advanced Reference:* Comprised of the five bones of the hand that connect the wrist (carpus) to the fingers (phalanges).

**Metals**  *Quick Reference:* Refers to the metals used in implants and medical devices, etc.
*Advanced Reference:* Metals which are used as implants; and are to enter the body require certain properties, i.e. insoluble, non-carcinogenic, non-toxic, non-irritant as well as possessing necessary strength as in the case of joints and plates. These include stainless steel, chrome, titanium, molybdenum, alloy and cobalt. Gold and silver could also be used, but cost alone excludes them.

**Metastasis**  *Quick Reference:* (met-ast-a-s-sees) Migration of disease from one area of the body to another.
  *Advanced Reference:* Generally used in relation to cancer spread from primary growth to secondary site.

**Metatarsals**  *Quick Reference:* Small bones of the foot.
  *Advanced Reference:* There are five in number and they run between the ankle and the toes.

**Methadone**  *Quick Reference:* Powerful narcotic analgesic.
  *Advanced Reference:* Used to relieve severe pain and in the treatment of heroin addiction.

**Methanol**  *Quick Reference:* Methyl alcohol. Better known as wood alcohol and used as a solvent.
  *Advanced Reference:* Much stronger than ***ethyl alcohol*** which comprises alcoholic drinks and if ingested can cause blindness and death. The blindness being due to damage to the optic nerve. Methylated spirit is a mixture of 5% methanol and 95% ethyl alcohol combined with other petroleum hydrocarbons. One form is known as surgical spirit or rubbing alcohol.

**Methicillin**  *Quick Reference:* Form of *penicillin.* A derivative of anti-staphylococcal or penicillinase-resistant penicillin.
  *Advanced Reference:* Main usage is in the treatment of penicillin-resistant *Staphylcoccus aureus.* Given only by injection.

**Methylene blue**  *Quick Reference:* (meth-il-ine) A blue dye.
  *Advanced Reference:* Used in staining material for microscopy and IV to test renal function and to identify various structures during surgery. Also used in the treatment of methaemoglobinaemia.

**Metoclopramide**  *Quick Reference:* An ***anti-emetic / anti-nauseant***. Also available as Maxolon and Primperan.
  *Advanced Reference:* Has a dual action whereby it acts centrally by depressing the *vomiting centre* and peripherally by stimulating gastro-intestinal emptying.

**Microbe**  *Quick Reference:* A micro-organism.
  *Advanced Reference:* More specifically a micro-organism capable of causing disease.

**Micturition**  *Quick Reference:* To make water.
  *Advanced Reference:* It is the act of passing urine.

**Midazolam**  *Quick Reference:* Drug used mainly for sedation.
  *Advanced Reference:* One of the ***benzodiazepine*** group of drugs. Used for premedication and induction of anaesthesia. Also known as *hypnovel.*

**Minihep**  *Quick Reference:* Proprietary anticoagulant.

*Advanced Reference:* Often used as subcutaneous injection for surgical patients to help prevent DVT.

**Minims**   *Quick Reference:* Proprietary **anticholinergic** drug.

*Advanced Reference:* Available in eye drop form as *atropine* sulphate. Used to dilate the pupils for purposes of ophthalmic examination.

**Miscarriage**   *Quick Reference:* The unexpected expulsion of the foetus before it is capable of sustaining independent life.

*Advanced Reference:* This period in the UK is generally seen as approximately 24–28 weeks. Sometimes used interchangeably with **abortion**.

**Mitral stenosis**   *Quick Reference:* Narrowing of the mitral valve.

*Advanced Reference:* Usually due to inflammation and caused by rheumatic fever. This leaves the valve shrunken and therefore leaks, reducing the efficiency of the heart generally.

**Mitral valve**   *Quick Reference:* Shaped like a mitre.

*Advanced Reference:* Also known as the bicuspid valve. Positioned between the left atrium and left ventricle of the heart.

**Mivacurium**   *Quick Reference: Non-depolarising* muscle relaxant.

*Advanced Reference:* Relatively short acting but with a slow onset of action. It is broken down by plasma (pseudo)-*cholinesterase* in the same way as *suxamethonium.*

**Mogadon**   *Quick Reference:* Tranquilliser and sedative drug.

*Advanced Reference:* Mogadon is a preparation of the long-acting *benzodiazepine*, nitrazepam.

**Molar**   *Quick Reference:* A back tooth.

*Advanced Reference:* Specifically indicates the double teeth, also referred to as grinders, of which there are three on either side of the jaw making a total of 12.

**Mole**   *Quick Reference:* A pigmented spot found on the skin.

*Advanced Reference:* Also refers to the amount in grams of a substance equal to its molecular weight. Mole indicates mass.

**Morbidity**   *Quick Reference:* Sickness rate.

*Advanced Reference:* Indicates the ratio of sick-to-well people in any given community.

**Morphine**   *Quick Reference:* (mor-feen) Narcotic analgesic.

*Advanced Reference:* An alkaloid of opium used to treat severe pain. May cause nausea and vomiting, reduces peristalsis. Used also as a premedication.

**Mortality**   *Quick Reference:* The ratio of deaths to the number of the population in a year.

*Advanced Reference:* Often expressed as deaths per thousand of the population. The mortality rate of a disease is the ratio of deaths from the disease to the total number of cases.

**Mouth gag**   *Quick Reference:* Anaesthetic adjunct used to open the mouth.
*Advanced reference:* A number of designs are available, the most commonly available being the Ferguson, which remains open due to a ratchet-type mechanism and the Mason's which contains a fixation screw to maintain the set degree of opening.

**MRI**   *Quick Reference:* Magnetic resonance imaging.
*Advanced Reference:* Imaging system used for diagnostic purposes, with many benefits over X-ray and computerised tomography (CT) scan. MRI provides an unparalleled view inside the body. It is the method of choice for the diagnosis of many types of injuries and conditions because of the ability to tailor the examination to the particular problem.

**MRSA**   *Quick Reference:* Methicillin-resistant *Staphylcoccus aureus.*
*Advanced Reference:* Involves bacteria (*Staphylcoccus aureus*) which have become resistant to the antibiotic **methicillin**, hence the term MRSA. At the present time, hospital acquired MRSA and associated deaths is increasing at alarming rates.

**Mucous membrane**   *Quick Reference:* Membrane that secretes mucus.
*Advanced Reference:* A layer of delicate skin-like tissue which contains glands that secrete mucous. Examples are the linings of the air passages and digestive tract, areas that have contact with the exterior.

**Multifocal**   *Quick Reference:* Term applied to abnormal heartbeat groupings.
*Advanced Reference:* Multifocal ectopic beats stem/originate from different focus areas of the heart. Also, multiformed indicates ectopic beats composed of more than one shape.

**Murmur**   *Quick Reference:* Heart sounds heard through a stethoscope in addition to the normal heart sounds.
*Advanced Reference:* These sounds may be due to vibrations and turbulence as the blood passes through the chambers and valves of the heart. Their presence does not necessarily indicate that disease is present.

**Muscle**   *Quick Reference:* The most abundant tissue in the human body. Responsible for various types of movement.
*Advanced Reference:* There are three types of muscle in the human body and differ in structure and function, namely *striated* (striped), *smooth* (involuntary) and *cardiac.*

**Muscle relaxant**   *Quick Reference:* Drug that prevents muscles contracting and so brings about relaxation.
*Advanced Reference:* For surgery, two main types are used: depolarising and non-depolarising which have differing actions at the neuromuscular end plate.

**Myocardial infarction**   *Quick Reference:* Result of a blockage of the blood supply to a part of the heart.

*Advanced Reference:* The blockage involves the coronary arteries and affects the myocardium causing mortification of the area insufficient in blood supply.

**Myocarditis**   *Quick Reference:* Inflammation of the heart muscle.

*Advanced Reference:* May be caused by a virus, bacteria or immunological reactions following infection.

**Myometrium**   *Quick Reference:* Muscular layer of the uterine wall.

*Advanced Reference:* Smooth muscle fibres of the myometrium curve around the uterus horizontally, vertically and diagonally.

**Myopia**   *Quick Reference:* Short sightedness.

*Advanced Reference:* Also referred to as near-sightedness. Involves changes to the focusing ability of the eye.

# N

**Naevus**  *Quick Reference:* (nevus) A birthmark.
*Advanced Reference:* Area of pigmentation on the skin due to dilated blood vessels.

**Nail brush**  *Quick Reference:* Small brush used during the scrub-up procedure.
*Advanced Reference:* Available as a pre-sterilised item and in some designs impregnated with antiseptic/antibacterial solution, etc. Not recommended by all authorities, some views are that too harsh a brush may cause skin injury and actually disturb resident flora and so create a better environment for bacterial growth. However, as originally intended for nail cleaning, has undoubted benefits.

**Naloxone**  *Quick Reference:* Opiate antagonist, e.g. narcan.
*Advanced Reference:* Used as an antidote to *narcotic* analgesic overdose.

**Nanogram**  *Quick Reference:* Indicates one-thousand millionth.
*Advanced Reference:* A nanogram is one-thousand millionth of a gram. A nanometre is one-thousand millionth of a metre. One-thousandth of a micron.

**Narcolepsy**  *Quick Reference:* A condition which produces an uncontrollable desire to sleep.
*Advanced Reference:* Those suffering the condition experience excessive daytime sleepiness and at the most inappropriate times.

**Narcosis**  *Quick Reference:* Dulling of consciousness.
*Advanced Reference:* A state of unconsciousness usually produced by drugs of the narcotic category.

**Narcotic**  *Quick Reference:* Any drug that produces narcosis.
*Advanced Reference:* Usually refers to morphine-type drugs. Other related terms are *opiates* and *opioids*.

**Nares**  *Quick Reference:* The nostrils.
*Advanced Reference:* The nares reach from the outside of the nose to the nasopharynx. The two nostrils are separated at the entrance by the collumella and within the nasal passages by the nasal septum.

**Nasal prongs/specs**  *Quick Reference:* Oxygen-delivery system.

*Advanced Reference:* Designed to be inserted one in each nostril for delivering oxygen. Inaccurate in percentage delivered as factors, such as depth of insertion, patient mouth opening, etc. have an effect. Values of 40% are quoted but cannot be taken as accurate. Claimed to deliver 4% for each 1 litre of $O^2$ flow, therefore a 6 litre $O^2$ flow would give 24% + 21% (room air) = 45%. A similar style with one nostril prong is also available. Often referred to as oxygen 'specs' due the design which loops over the top of the ears.

**Nasogastric tube**  *Quick Reference:* Tube (usually polyvinyl chloride, PVC) passed into the stomach.

*Advanced Reference:* Usually inserted for suction, lavage or feeding. Available in a number of bores, e.g. 10G through 18G, etc. Also referred to as Ryles tube, which is a nasogastric tube with a weighted tip. It has an integral radio-opaque line for placement detection by X-ray when *in situ*. In order to maintain some degree of rigidity, they are often kept in the department fridge.

**Nasopharyngeal airway**  *Quick Reference:* Airway used primarily in anaesthesia.

*Advanced Reference:* Inserted via the nostrils and sits in the pharynx. Available in various diameters from neonate to large adult. Lengths also vary accordingly and may be assessed by comparing the distance from nares to ear.

**Nasopharynx**  *Quick Reference:* Region behind the nose.

*Advanced Reference:* The nasopharynx is actually the upper pharynx, the portion above and behind the soft palate.

**Nausea**  *Quick Reference:* Sensation of being about to vomit.

*Advanced Reference:* Actually indicates the feeling of sickness without vomiting actually occurring.

**Navel**  *Quick Reference:* The umbilicus.

*Advanced Reference:* The scar in the centre of the abdominal wall where the umbilical cord joined the foetus to the *placenta* in the *womb*.

**Nebuliser**  *Quick Reference:* Device that converts a liquid into a fine spray.

*Advanced Reference:* Apparatus for administering a drug in the form of a spray, cloud or droplets. Also used to humidify inspired oxygen or gases. Also referred to as an atomiser.

**Necrosis**  *Quick Reference:* Death of an organ or portion of it.

*Advanced Reference:* Usually caused by damage or interruption to the blood supply or because of bacterial infection.

**Needle holder**  *Quick Reference:* Instrument for holding sutures/needles during surgery.

*Advanced Reference:* Available in various designs and sizes depending on need and speciality. Examples are Mayo, Gillies, Castroviejo, Crile-wood, Kilner, Debakey.

**Needle-stick injury**   *Quick Reference:* Injury from a hypodermic needle.

*Advanced Reference:* Refers to stabbing with a hypodermic needle or similar used in clinical areas. Can be a route of cross infection and due to its potential seriousness many policies and devices have been introduced in an attempt to lower incidence.

**Needle valve**   *Quick Reference:* Control mechanism on a flowmeter, such as oxygen, nitrous oxide, on an anaesthetic machine.

*Advanced Reference:* They increase or decrease the flow of gas as it is turned clockwise or anti-clockwise.

**Neomycin**   *Quick Reference:* Broad-spectrum antibiotic.

*Advanced Reference:* Effective against topical bacteria. Too toxic to be used intravenously (IV) or intramuscularly (IM).

**Neonatal**   *Quick Reference:* Of newborn baby, neonate.

*Advanced Reference:* Conventionally used to indicate the first 4 weeks of life.

**Neoplasm**   *Quick Reference:* New growth or tumour.

*Advanced Reference:* A *tumour* that may be *benign* or *malignant*.

**Neostigmine**   *Quick Reference:* An anticholinesterase drug.

*Advanced Reference:* Increases the activity of the neurotransmitter *acetylcholine*, which transmits instructions from the brain to skeletal muscle. Used as a reversal to non-depolarising muscle relaxants.

**Nephrectomy**   *Quick Reference:* Surgical removal of the *kidney*.

*Advanced Reference:* Removal of one or both kidneys due to various diseases and conditions.

**Nephritis**   *Quick Reference:* Inflammation of the kidneys.

*Advanced Reference:* A non-specific term that may be used to describe a wide variety of diseases of the kidney.

**Nephrostomy**   *Quick Reference:* Draining of the kidney directly to the exterior.

*Advanced Reference:* Involves the insertion of a self-retaining catheter through a small incision in the cortex. The commonest reason for this procedure is bilateral ureteric obstruction.

**Nerve**   *Quick Reference:* A bundle of conducting fibres.

*Advanced Reference:* Nerve fibres are contained in a sheath of connective tissue which run from the central nervous system (*CNS*) to the muscles, skin and other organs conveying either motor or sensory impulses. The nervous system is divided into *CNS*, which includes the brain and spinal cord, the *peripheral nervous system* and the *autonomic system* which comprises the sympathetic and parasympathetic systems.

N

**Nerve block** *Quick Reference:* Indicates blocking nerve pathways to prevent pain.

*Advanced Reference:* Carried out using local anaesthetic (LA) agents. Examples are *wound infiltration* (following surgery), *digital block* (provides pain relief following surgery on toes and fingers), *intercostal block* (carried out for rib fractures or following surgery), *femoral block* (useful in patients with fractured neck of femur) or *ankle block* (following surgery). In addition to LAs for this purpose, electrical nerve stimulation, acupuncture, cryotherapy as well as drugs and inhalation agents are all used as pain-blocking techniques.

**Nerve stimulator** *Quick Reference:* Peripheral stimulator used to assess neuromuscular blockade with muscle relaxants.

*Advanced Reference:* Used to monitor transmission across the neuromuscular junction with reference to reversal of muscle relaxants. Also used during nerve blocks to produce muscular contractions when locating a nerve plexus.

**Neurofibroma** *Quick Reference:* Benign tumour.

*Advanced Reference:* A benign tumour arising from the sheath of a nerve.

**Neuroleptic** *Quick Reference:* (nuro-lep-tic) Drug which effects the nervous system in the way of quietening emotional behaviour and slowing psychomotor activity.

*Advanced Reference:* Term applied to a technique of anaesthesia which involves using opioid analgesics such as fentanyl and phenoperidine in combination with, e.g. droperidol. Produces neurolepsis and a reduction in motor activity.

**Neuroma** *Quick Reference:* A tumour consisting of nerve fibres.

*Advanced Reference:* A tumour growing from a nerve.

**Neurons** *Quick Reference:* Or neurones. Nerve cell.

*Advanced Reference:* A nerve cell with conducting fibres.

**Nifedipine** *Quick Reference:* A calcium antagonist. Antihypertensive.

*Advanced Reference:* Used in the treatment of hypotension and angina.

**Nikethamide** *Quick Reference:* Respiratory-stimulant drug.

*Advanced Reference:* Used to relieve severe respiratory difficulties, e.g. respiratory depression, chronic respiratory disease.

**Nipple** *Quick Reference:* Projection at the top of the breast.

*Advanced Reference:* Structure through which a baby/offspring withdraws milk.

**Nipride** *Quick Reference:* Proprietary form of the antihypertensive drug sodium nitroprusside.

*Advanced Reference:* Used to treat high blood pressure (BP) and create hypotension during surgery by vasodilatation. Short acting. Used in theatres as a preparation for reconstitution in 5% dextrose. Should be protected from light as it decomposes to form unstable solutions which may lead to cyanide toxicity.

**Nitric oxide**   *Quick Reference:* Chemical symbol NO.
*Advanced Reference:* Used in intensive care units (ICUs), etc. in inhalant form as a pulmonary vasodilator.

**Nitrogen**   *Quick Reference:* Inert colourless gas.
*Advanced Reference:* Present at a level of 78% in air. Not able to support life but plays a part in supporting the alveoli of the lungs.

**Nitrous oxide**   *Quick Reference:* Laughing gas, $N_2O$.
*Advanced Reference:* Weak analgesic and anaesthetic. Given in combination with oxygen during general anaesthesia. Available as a compressed liquid in blue cylinders.

**Node**   *Quick Reference:* (or nodule) A protuberance or swelling.
*Advanced Reference:* Various nodes exist throughout the body, e.g. atrioventricular (*AV*) *node* and *sino-atrial node* in the heart which are responsible for impulse transmission. The nodes of Ranvier are present in nerve fibres. Also *lymph nodes*.

**Nodule**   *Quick Reference:* A small swelling.
*Advanced Reference:* A small mass of rounded or irregular shape. As a tumour growth or calcification near an arthritic joint.

**Non-depolariser**   *Quick Reference:* Refers to a specific group of muscle relaxants which act at the neuromuscular junction.
*Advanced Reference:* These drugs attach themselves to receptor sites on the post-synaptic membrane of the neuromuscular junction and prevent acetylcholine reaching the end plate and producing depolarisation. Whereas depolarising muscle relaxants produce their effect (prolonged contraction and paralysis) at the membrane in the same way as acetylcholine.

**Non-invasive**   *Quick Reference:* Indicates not entering inside the body.
*Advanced Reference:* As opposed to invasive, when devices, etc. are placed inside the body. An example is non-invasive BP using a limb cuff as opposed to cannulating an artery to obtain a direct recording.

**Non-rebreathing**   *Quick Reference:* Refers to valves used in breathing systems.
*Advanced Reference:* With these circuits the patient continually receives a fresh flow of gas. Examples in common use are Ruben valve and those as used in bagvalve mask (BVM) devices for resuscitation.

**Non-steroidal anti-inflammatory drugs**   *Quick Reference:* NSAID. Group of drugs with analgesic, anti-inflammatory and antipyretic actions.

*Advanced Reference:* Thought to act by inhibiting *prostaglandin* synthesis and so decreasing the inflammatory response to surgery, etc. and associated pain. Commonly used examples are *diclofenac* and *ketorolac*. On a basic level *aspirin* is also a member of this group.

**Noradrenaline** *Quick Reference:* A catecholamine, hormone secreted by the medulla of the adrenal glands.

*Advanced Reference:* Closely related to adrenaline but not as selective in its actions. A neurotransmitter of the sympathetic nervous system. Noradrenaline is almost entirely concerned with contraction of the arteries and supporting BP.

**Normal saline** *Quick Reference:* Indicates an isotonic solution of sodium chloride. Normal is in terms of physiological rather than in chemistry where this represents a totally different strength.

*Advanced Reference:* An isotonic solution of sodium chloride is 0.9%. Used as an IV maintenance and replacement fluid as well as a vehicle for medications.

**Normasol** *Quick Reference:* Proprietary saline solution.

*Advanced Reference:* Produced in the form of a sterile solution and used to clean burns and minor wounds. Also available in ophthalmic form as an eye wash.

**Normothermic/normothermia** *Quick Reference:* (nor-mo-ther-mic) The presence of normal body temperature.

*Advanced Reference:* When the core body temperature is between 36.5°C and 37.2°C (approximately).

**Nose** *Quick Reference:* Organ of smell and air passage.

*Advanced Reference:* Air is drawn from the exterior via the two nostrils which are separated by the septum, and warmed, humidified and filtered before progressing to the respiratory tract. The lower septum is comprised of cartilage and the upper part of bone. The *olfactory* nerve conveys sense of smell to the brain.

**Nosocomial** *Quick Reference:* Infections that are acquired during hospitalisation.

*Advanced Reference:* Acquired from either patient or staff source. Includes bacterial and fungal infections and may be due to an already reduced resistance.

**Nosworthy** *Quick Reference:* (nose-worthy) Type of endotracheal (ET) tube connector.

*Advanced Reference:* Of metal design and now replaced by the standard fitting which are made from plastic/PVC.

**Noxyflex** *Quick Reference:* A proprietary microbial agent.

*Advanced Reference:* Produced in the form of a powder for reconstitution and often used for wound and cavity washout.

**Nubain**   *Quick Reference:* Narcotic analgesic drug.

*Advanced Reference:* Used to treat moderate to severe pain. A preparation of the opiate namely *nalbuphine*.

**Nystagmus**   *Quick Reference:* (ni-stig-mus) Involuntary eyeball movement.

*Advanced Reference:* Both side-to-side and, less commonly, up-and-down movement are involved or a combination of both when a rotary movement occurs. May be due to CNS disease.

**Obesity**   *Quick Reference:* Excess of fat in the body.

*Advanced Reference:* Excessive amount of fat throughout the body, which can be calculated by using body mass index (***BMI***) formula.

**Oblique**   *Quick Reference:* Indicates slanting, declining from the vertical or horizontal, diverging from a straight line.

*Advanced Reference:* Used in regard to muscles. The muscles in the wall of the abdomen which slant from side to centre. The two muscles which are responsible for turning the eye upwards/downwards and inwards/outwards.

**Obstetrics**   *Quick Reference:* Medical care in pregnancy and childbirth.

*Advanced Reference:* Involves both midwifery and an obstetric and gynaecological specialist doctor.

**Obstruction**   *Quick Reference:* Common term used in relation to anaesthetics and surgery.

*Advanced Reference:* With reference to surgery can indicate intestinal obstruction, which can be due to a number of causes, e.g. tumour, twisting, strangulation, etc. while in anaesthesia indicates obstruction of the airway and can be at any level; examples can include, lips, tongue, blood, vomit, foreign body, etc. The term could also be used to describe obstructions in patient breathing systems.

**Obtund**   *Quick Reference:* To deaden pain. To blunt.

*Advanced Reference:* To render insensitive to painful stimuli by reducing the level of consciousness as in anaesthesia or with the use of opioid analgesics.

**Obturator**   *Quick Reference:* Something which occludes an opening.

*Advanced Reference:* Obturator nerve block targets the obturator nerve which supplies the muscles of the thigh/hip. Also, an *oesophageal obturator airway* has two lumens, of which one is occluded and is intended to block the oesophagus and therefore leave the trachea available.

**Occipital**   *Quick Reference:* Indicates the back of the head.

*Advanced Reference:* The occipital bone is the back of the floor of the skull and forms a moveable joint with the spine. The brain stem passes through a hole in the occipital bone and becomes the spinal cord. The occipital lobe of the brain is at the back of the skull above the *cerebellum*, it records and interprets vision.

**Occult**   *Quick Reference:* Concealed, cut off from view.

*Advanced Reference:* Occult blood refers to blood that is not evident to the naked eye. Common example is blood in stools which is not visible but can be detected through laboratory examinations.

**ODP**   *Quick Reference:* Operating Department Practitioner.

*Advanced Reference:* Professional that works alongside surgeons and anaesthetists, and trained for general theatre work. Previous titles in the development of the discipline included Operating Department Assistant (ODA) and Theatre Technician.

**Oedema**   *Quick Reference:* Swelling due to the accumulation of excess tissue fluid.

*Advanced Reference:* May be due to local causes such as interference with *lymphatic* or venous drainage or generalised conditions such as heart or *kidney* failure. *Pulmonary oedema* is the accumulation of fluid in the lungs. Oedematous indicates an area affected by oedema.

**Oesophageal obturator**   *Quick Reference:* A type of oral airway with an attached *face mask*.

*Advanced Reference:* Used when *intubation* with endotracheal (ET) tube is not possible and at emergency resuscitation, etc.; these devices are designed to be inserted blindly with the intention of entering the oesophagus, blocking it off, thus allowing for tracheal ventilation with *oxygen* from a second lumen which opens higher up the tube. A number of designs are in existence, all varying slightly in working principle and it is this point that has hindered their popularity. However, they are in common use by paramedics in some countries such as the USA.

**Oesophageal stethoscope**   *Quick Reference:* Multi-lumen device which is placed in the oesophagus during anaesthesia.

*Advanced Reference:* Disposable tube placed in the oesophagus, as with a *nasogastric tube*, which has lumens for attaching a *stethoscope* and temperature probe.

**Oesophagectomy**   *Quick Reference:* Surgical removal of part or whole of the oesophagus.

*Advanced Reference:* May be performed for certain conditions of the oesophagus, e.g. carcinoma. Often combined with a partial or total *gastrectomy*.

**Oesophago-gastrectomy**   *Quick Reference:* Removal of part of oesophagus and stomach.

*Advanced Reference:* Excision of the lower third of the oesophagus and all of the stomach, usually carried out due to tumours at or near the oesophago-gastric junction. An anastomosis is made between the jejunum and oesophagus.

**Oesophagoscopy**   *Quick Reference:* Examination of the oesophagus with an oesophagoscope.

*Advanced Reference:* Originally an oesophagoscope was a rigid instrument with an attached light source; however, flexible scopes with built-in fibre light sources have more or less replaced the rigid variety.

**Oesophagus**   *Quick Reference:* Food canal, gullet.

*Advanced Reference:* The oesophagus extends from the *pharynx* to the *stomach*, passing through the chest and diaphragm. In the adult is approximately 23–25 cm long.

**Oestrogen**   *Quick Reference:* (east-ro-gen) Female sex *hormone*.

*Advanced Reference:* Oestradiol is the hormone naturally secreted by the female ovaries and any substance which has a similar action to this hormone is called an *oestrogen*. Oestrogens are involved in the development of the secondary sexual characteristics at puberty, stimulation of menstruation and suppression of ovulation. They may be natural or synthetic, are used in the contraceptive pill and for treating certain menstrual disorders. Oestrogens are associated with an increased risk of intravascular clotting.

**Ohm**   *Quick Reference:* SI unit of electrical resistance.

*Advanced Reference:* Ohm's law involves the resistance of a current passing through a conductor:

voltage = current (amperes) × resistance (Ohms) or

with reference to the flow of fluids;

pressure = flow × resistance.

**Olecranon**   *Quick Reference:* Upper end of the ulna bone.
*Advanced Reference:* Forms the point or prominence of the elbow.

**Olfactory**   *Quick Reference:* Concerned with the sense of smell.

*Advanced Reference:* The olfactory nerve conveys the sensations of smell from the nose to the brain. It is the first cranial nerve and runs from the upper part of the nose through the *ethmoid* bone and into the brain. Injury or disease to this nerve causes a loss of smell.

**Oliguria**   *Quick Reference:* Diminished flow of urine.

*Advanced Reference:* May be due to severe dehydration or renal failure.

**Omentum**   *Quick Reference:* Apron of peritoneum which hangs from the *stomach* and *colon* to lie in front of the intestines.

O

*Advanced Reference:* Referred to as the abdominal policeman as it may adhere to inflamed areas in an attempt to separate them off from the rest of the abdominal cavity. There are in fact two sections of the omentum; *greater*, which hangs from the greater curvature of the stomach in front of the intestine and the *lesser*, which is attached to the lesser curvature of the stomach and attaches the stomach to the undersurface of the *liver*.

**Oncology**   *Quick Reference:* The study of malignant tumours.
*Advanced Reference:* An oncologist is a specialist in the diagnosis and treatment of cancer. Also given as a second title to surgeons who deal with cancer treatment within their specific surgical speciality.

**Ondansetron**   *Quick Reference:* Anti-emetic drug.
*Advanced Reference:* Developed to treat the severe nausea associated with chemotherapy. Often given preoperatively then at intervals during and after surgery. Most commonly known by the proprietary name, *zofran*.

**One-lung anaesthesia**   *Quick Reference:* Anaesthetic technique used in thoracic surgery.
*Advanced Reference:* Involves the deliberate collapse of one lung using a bronchial blocker or endobronchial (ET) tube, usually to improve surgical access.

**Oopherectomy**   *Quick Reference:* Removal of one or both ovaries.
*Advanced Reference:* Oophor(o)- is a prefix indicating the ovaries. Oophoropexy is the surgical fixation to the pelvic wall of a displaced ovary. An oophorosalpingectomy is the removal of an ovary and its associated uterine (fallopian) tube.

**Opacity**   *Quick Reference:* Pertaining to an opaque quality.
*Advanced Reference:* An opaque substance neither transmits nor allows passage of light. Neither transparent or translucent. A cataract is an opacity of the lens of the eye.

**Operating theatre**   *Quick Reference:* Area of a hospital where surgery is carried out.
*Advanced Reference:* Referred to simply as theatre. In some countries the term operating room or OR is used. Operating theatres indicates a suite of ORs or areas rather than implying the singular.

**Operidine**   *Quick Reference:* A proprietary narcotic analgesic.
*Advanced Reference:* Operidine is a preparation of phenoperidine. Used primarily as an analgesic during surgery.

**Ophthalmic**   *Quick Reference:* Relating to the eye.
*Advanced Reference:* Ophthalmology indicates medical and surgical care of the eyes. An *ophthalmologist* is a medical practitioner specialising

in this work. An *ophthalmoscope* is an illuminated instrument used for examining the interior of the eye.

**Opiate**   *Quick Reference:* A ***narcotic*** drug.
*Advanced Reference:* Indicates a drug that is derived from opium, e.g. ***morphine***.

**Orbit**   *Quick Reference:* Bony cavity containing the eyeball.
*Advanced Reference:* The orbit is made up parts of eight bones.

**Orchidectomy**   *Quick Reference:* Removal of one or both testicles.
*Advanced Reference:* The testicles are referred to as orchids. The prefix orchi(o)- indicates the testis or of the testicles. Orchitis is inflammation of the testis.

**Orchidopexy**   *Quick Reference:* It is fixation of the testis into the scrotum.
*Advanced Reference:* Commonly carried out because of torsion of the testis or to prevent it happening if there is a potential risk.

**Organ donation**   *Quick Reference:* Refers to giving a body organ for transplantation. Many members of the UK public carry donor cards indicating their willingness for organs to be used for transplantation in the event of their death. Some countries operate a system directly opposite to this arrangement where organs may be taken unless objection to removal has been specifically stated.
*Advanced Reference:* Usually involves hearts, lungs, kidneys, liver and cornea. Donation can be from both *live* and ***cadaver*** sources. The term harvesting is used when a number of organs are to be retrieved from a cadaver. Organs such as a kidney donated by a living relative are termed '***live-related donors***.'

**Organ of Corti**   *Quick Reference:* The true organ of hearing.
*Advanced Reference:* The organ of Corti is situated within the membranous labyrinth of the cochlea.

**Orifice**   *Quick Reference:* An opening.
*Advanced Reference:* Can be applied to a number of bodily openings, e.g. mouth, anus and ear.

**Oropharyngeal**   *Quick Reference:* (oro-farin-geal) Indicates approaching or entering the ***pharynx*** via the oral cavity.
*Advanced Reference:* Term used with reference to airways. Oropharyngeal is an airway placed in the mouth reaching back into the pharynx and a ***Nasopharyngeal*** airway is an airway placed in one nostril and reaches back into the pharynx. Assessment of length measurement is from the ear to corner of the mouth.

**Oropharynx**   *Quick Reference:* (oro-farinx) The lower part of the pharynx.
*Advanced Reference:* Situated below the nasopharynx, behind the tongue.

**Orthopaedics**   *Quick Reference:* Bones, joints and muscles.

*Advanced Reference:* Orthopaedics is the branch of surgery related to disease, injuries and distortion of the bones, joints and muscles. The word *orthopaedics* itself means *straight children*.Going back to the time when children suffered with rickettes, the main aim then, was to straighten their bones.

**Orthopnoea**   *Quick Reference:* Breathing with relation to body position, i.e. unless in an upright position.

*Advanced Reference:* Refers to when a patient may have difficulty in breathing when laying flat, etc. Seen in patients with heart and lung conditions.

**Oscilloscope**   *Quick Reference:* Apparatus which displays recorded signals usually on a screen.

*Advanced Reference:* Regular use is made of oscilloscopes with electro-cardiographical (ECG) reading and recording.

**Oscillotonometer**   *Quick Reference:* Apparatus used to indirectly record blood pressure (BP).

*Advanced Reference:* A non-invasive method of reading BP. The Von Recklinghausen oscillotonometer consists of a double cuff, one to occlude the artery and the other, a sensing cuff, attached to an inflating bulb and reading dial. Following inflation, slow release of pressure allows for deflections of the oscillating needle as systolic and diastolic pressures to kick in and record a reading.

**Osmolality**   *Quick Reference:* Expression of concentration of active particles in solution.

*Advanced Reference:* Osmolality is the number of osmoles per kilogram solvent.

**Osmosis**   *Quick Reference:* Selective migration of molecules through semipermeable membranes.

*Advanced Reference:* The passage of fluid from a low-concentration solution to one of a higher concentration through a semipermeable membrane. Osmotic pressure refers to the pressure exerted by large molecules such as globulin proteins in the blood which assist in drawing fluid into the circulation from surrounding tissues.

**Osseous**   *Quick Reference:* Pertaining to bone.

*Advanced Reference:* Consisting of or resembling bone.

**Ossicles**   *Quick Reference:* Small bones of the middle ear.

*Advanced Reference:* The ossicles comprise of the malleus, incus and stapes, all involved in the relay of sound waves.

**Osteo-**   *Quick Reference:* Refers to bone, a prefix.

*Advanced Reference:* Used as a prefix when referring to a bone condition/procedure in medicine(*osteotomy*).

**Osteotomy**    *Quick Reference:* A surgical operation of cutting a bone.
*Advanced Reference:* Cutting into or through a bone. May be performed to correct a deformity.

**Otitis media**    *Quick Reference:* Inflammation of the middle ear.
*Advanced Reference:* Due to infection within the ear drum which commonly arises in the back of the nose and reaches the ear via the *eustachian tube*.

**Otorrhoea**    *Quick Reference:* (ot-or-ea) A watery discharge from the ear.
*Advanced Reference:* A discharge from the ear often caused by an ear infection (*otitis media*).

**Otrivine**    *Quick Reference:* A proprietary nasal decongestant.
*Advanced Reference:* A sympathomimetic in the form of drops and spray which may be used during nasal surgery.

**Ouabaine**    *Quick Reference:* (u-bane) Proprietary heart-stimulant drug.
*Advanced Reference:* Used to treat various forms of heart attack, heart failure and sever heartbeat irregularity.

**Oval window**    *Quick Reference:* Oval-shaped aperture in the wall of the middle ear.
*Advanced Reference:* Leads to the inner ear.

**Ovaries**    *Quick Reference:* Female sex glands.
*Advanced Reference:* Two almond-shaped glands, situated in the pelvis in the female body. They are responsible for producing ova which pass down the fallopian tubes into the uterus and hormones which help control the menstrual cycle.

**Oxford**    *Quick Reference:* Refers to a number of anaesthetic-related adjuncts.
*Advanced Reference:* There is an oxford ventilator, tracheal tube, airway, vaporiser and infant laryngoscope blade.

**Oxidation**    *Quick Reference:* Rust is a form of oxidation.
*Advanced Reference:* Combination of a substance with oxygen.

**Oximeter**    *Quick Reference:* A piece of monitoring equipment used to determine the oxygen saturation of the blood.
*Advanced Reference:* The oximeter probe can be attached to an ear or finger to measure the level of oxygen saturation in the blood. Usually available as a pulse-oximeter which have the facility for providing both pulse rate and oxygen saturation.

**Oxygen**   *Quick Reference:* A colourless, odourless gas necessary to support life.

*Advanced Reference:* Oxygen is essential for life. It is transported to the tissues from the lungs in combination with the blood pigment haemoglobin.

**Oxygen bypass**   *Quick Reference:* System for direct oxygen delivery built into anaesthetic machines.

*Advanced Reference:* Arrangement for bypassing oxygen delivery from going through the flowmeters to direct delivery via the fresh gas flow (FGF) route, usually by operation of a push-button or trigger mounted conveniently on the anaesthetic machine.

**Oxygen failure device**   *Quick Reference:* Device fitted into anaesthetic machines.

*Advanced Reference:* Similar ideas and early versions were referred to as a Bowsons whistle. Although differing in function, the intention remains to provide an audible warning when oxygen availability and delivery to the patient fails.

**Oxyhaemoglobin**   *Quick Reference:* Haemoglobin which has been oxygenated.

*Advanced Reference:* Oxygenation of haemoglobin is present in arterial blood and deoxygenated in venous blood.

**Oxytocin**   *Quick Reference:* A hormone of the pituitary gland.

*Advanced Reference:* Oxytocin stimulates contraction of the uterus which is especially sensitive to its action towards the end of pregnancy. Used to institute contractions of the uterus, if labour is delayed.

**Ozone**   *Quick Reference:* Form of oxygen.

*Advanced Reference:* Ozone has three atoms instead of two ($O_3$).

# P

**Packed red cells**   *Quick Reference:* Intravenous (IV) blood product.
*Advanced Reference:* Also termed **plasma**-reduced blood. It is whole blood with a volume of plasma removed which is then used in the production of alternative blood products.

**Pallor**   *Quick Reference:* Unusual paleness of the skin.
*Advanced Reference:* Caused by a reduced flow of blood or deficiency in normal pigments.

**Palmer**   *Quick Reference:* Relating to the palm of the hand.
*Advanced Reference:* Also the palmer arches which indicates the **anastomosis** of the *radial* and *ulna* arteries in the hand.

**Palmer fasciectomy**   *Quick Reference:* (fas-she-ec-tommy) Operation to remove abnormal, thickened tissue in the palm.
*Advanced Reference:* Also known as **Dupuytren's** *contracture*. The condition is produced by a progressive thickening and contraction of the palmer aponeurosis resulting in flexion of the ring, middle and little fingers. *Excision* of abnormal tissue (fasciectomy) allows return of finger movement.

**Palpate**   *Quick Reference:* To palpate, to feel, with the hands. Palpation.
*Advanced Reference:* Examination via the surface of the body of the position, size and shape of internal organs.

**Pan**   *Quick Reference:* All.
*Advanced Reference:* Examples are *pandemic* (affecting all of the population), *pan-procto-colectomy* (removal of all of the colon).

**Panadol**   *Quick Reference:* Painkiller.
*Advanced Reference:* Alternative name *paracetamol*. It has similar action to *aspirin* but has no anti-inflammatory action. It is used in preference to aspirin with children.

**Pancreas**   *Quick Reference:* Large **gland** situated across the back wall of the upper abdominal cavity behind the stomach.
*Advanced Reference:* A dual purpose gland which forms part of the digestive system. Its **exocrine** secretions help to neutralise acid while

P

its *endocrine* secretion; *insulin,* passes directly into the bloodstream and is involved in the chemical control of sugar in the body.

**Pancuronium**   *Quick Reference:* Non-depolarising muscle relaxant.
*Advanced Reference:* Alternative name is *Pavulon.* A synthetic non-depolarising muscle relaxant with an approximate duration of action of 30 min. May produce slight *tachycardia* and rise in *blood pressure* (BP). Not thought to cause histamine release and does not cross the placenta in significant amounts. Metabolised in the liver.

**PaO$_2$**   *Quick Reference:* Symbol for arterial oxygen level.
*Advanced Reference:* Partial pressure of $O_2$ in arterial blood.

**Papaveretum**   *Quick Reference:* (pa-pav-er-ertum) Compound preparation of alkaloids of opium, e.g. *omnopon.*
*Advanced Reference:* Comprised of mainly morphine plus *codeine,* noscapine and *papaverine.* Used as a narcotic analgesic for both pre-medication and post-operative pain relief.

**Papaverine**   *Quick Reference:* A smooth muscle relaxant.
*Advanced Reference:* It is technically an *opiate* but possesses little or no *analgesic* effect. Used in the treatment of *bronchospasm* in *asthma.* Used with relation to theatres in vascular surgery to relax vessel ends for *anastomosis* and to relax an artery after inadvertent injection which has caused spasm.

**Para**   *Quick Reference:* Next to or to the side of.
*Advanced Reference:* Examples are *paramedian* (incision)(situated to the side of the midline), *paramedical* (professions and services working alongside the medical sciences), etc.

**Paraldehyde**   *Quick Reference:* Fast-acting sedative.
*Advanced Reference:* Used in the treatment of severe and continuous epileptic seizures. Administered by injection but may be given rectally. Recognised by its distinctive strong smell.

**Paraphimosis**   *Quick Reference:* (para-fi-mosis) Tight foreskin.
*Advanced Reference:* Occurs when a tight foreskin is drawn back behind the glans of the penis and swelling or engorgement prevents replacement. If persistent a *circumcision* is performed.

**Parasite**   *Quick Reference:* Creature that lives at the expense of another.
*Advanced Reference:* In humans most parasites have the potential to cause illness. These can include *viruses, bacteria, fungi, protozoa* and *worms.*

**Parathyroidectomy**   *Quick Reference:* Surgical removal of the *parathyroid glands.*

*Advanced Reference:* Carried out because of hyperparathyroidism, when usually all four glands are removed. Overactivity causes an increased level of calcium in the blood which can result in stone formation in the renal tract.

**Parathyroid glands**   *Quick Reference:* Group of small yellow-coloured glands situated behind or attached to the thyroid glands.

*Advanced Reference:* Their function is to secrete the hormone parathormone which regulates the use of calcium in the body. If the blood concentration of calcium falls, the parathyroids are stimulated to produce more of the hormone and this increases the solubility of calcium in the bones and restores the blood levels to normal. Overactivity or stimulation of the parathyroids is often due to a tumour, may produce an excess of parathormone and consequently too much calcium is then withdrawn from the bones and they become fragile. The surplus calcium is excreted in the urine and can lead to kidney stones. If the condition warrants it, surgical removal is usually carried out sometimes involving splitting of the sternum.

**Parenteral**   *Quick Reference:* Indicates outside of or away from *enteral* route. Not via mouth or bowel.

*Advanced Reference: Total parenteral nutrition (**TPN**)* indicates a feeding process other than the alimentary route (enteral). TPN involves intravenous (IV) feeding for patients unable to take food orally or absorb in the gut due to disease, surgery, etc.

**Parietal**   *Quick Reference:* (par-e-atal) Indicates the inner walls of a body cavity.

*Advanced Reference:* Common example is the parietal *pleura,* which is attached to the chest wall.

**Parotid**   *Quick Reference:* Salivary gland situated just in front of the ear and the angle of the lower jaw.

*Advanced Reference:* It has a duct which opens into the mouth. Can become enlarged by inflammation, infection or presence of a stone.

**Pascal**   *Quick Reference:* The SI unit for pressure. Abrreviated as Pa.

*Advanced Reference:* Due to small size of the pascal, pressure is usually measured in kilopascals. Bar and mercury (mmHg) are also used to measure pressure. 1 atmosphere (atm) = 760 mmHg = 1 bar = 100,000 Pa = 100 kPa = 15 lb/in.$^2$.

**Passive**   *Quick Reference:* Indicates inactivity.

*Advanced Reference:* An example to theatres could be *passive-scavenging system* which involved expired gases diverting to container where volatile agents adhered to carbon/charcoal granules.

**Pasteurisation**   *Quick Reference:* (past-your-isa-shon) Disinfection process.
*Advanced Reference:* Involves the use of heat (hot water) at a temperature of between 60°C and 80°C. Not a sterilising process. Used for surgical instruments, rigid scopes, anaesthetic equipments, etc.

**Patch test**   *Quick Reference:* Skin test for identifying allergies.
*Advanced Reference:* Allergies, such as those due to food, pollen, animal fur, etc. but can be used for chemicals, such as skin preps, etc.

**Patent**   *Quick Reference:* Open, clear.
*Advanced Reference:* Not occluded. As with vessels such as fallopian tubes and blood vessels.

**Pathogenic**   *Quick Reference:* A disease-producing agent.
*Advanced Reference:* Pathogenic organisms are capable of causing disease.

**Patties**   *Quick Reference:* Small swab used in neurosurgery.
*Advanced Reference:* Small piece of lint with a length of cotton attached. Usually used wet to absorb blood and to cover and delicate exposed tissue during craniotomy.

**PCA**   *Quick Reference:* Patient-controlled analgesia.
*Advanced Reference:* System in which the small doses of analgesic, sometimes combined with an anti-emetic, are administered by the patient themselves as and when required, usually into the post-operative period. This involves an infusion device pre-programmed to deliver set doses in increment form or as boluses. The machines also have many safety aspects designed to avoid overdosage.

**PEG tube**   *Quick Reference:* Percutaneous endoscopic gastrostomy tube.
*Advanced Reference:* Feeding tube inserted directly into the stomach and used when patients are unable to take nutrition orally due to various conditions.

**Pelvis**   *Quick Reference:* Lower limb girdle composed of the lower part of the backbone and the two hip bones.
*Advanced Reference:* The pelvis is the large complex of bones shaped like a basin and connects the spine with the legs and contains the lower part of the abdominal cavity. It is composed of the two hip bones, namely *sacrum* and the *coccyx*. In front the two hip bones meet at the *symphysis pubis* and behind they join the sacrum.

**Penbritin**   *Quick Reference:* Broad-spectrum antibiotic.
*Advanced Reference:* Proprietary form of ampicillin. Used to treat respiratory infections and those of the urinary tract and middle ear.

**Penicillin**   *Quick Reference:* First **antibiotic** to be used.
*Advanced Reference:* First reported use in 1941. There are now many closely related antibiotics which are compounds of *aminopenicillanic acid*. The acid itself being first extracted from moulds.

**Pentaspan**   *Quick Reference:* Pentastarch. Synthetic **colloid**.
*Advanced Reference:* Plasma expander that increases plasma volume by 1.5 times. Does not interfere with clotting as with some alternatives.

**Penthrane**   *Quick Reference:* Volatile anaesthetic agent.
*Advanced Reference:* Now withdrawn mainly due to its potential toxic effects on the kidneys.

**Peptic (ulcer)**   *Quick Reference:* Ulceration in either **stomach** or **duodenum**.
*Advanced Reference:* Causes include; overproduction of acid and pepsin, stress, etc.

**Percutaneous**   *Quick Reference:* Per means through, by way of; cutaneous, means pertaining to the skin.
*Advanced Reference:* Indicates to pass through the skin in order to reach an inner area for treatment, e.g. percutaneous lithotripsy.

**Perfuse/sion**   *Quick Reference:* Passage of a liquid through body tissues or an organ.
*Advanced Reference:* Tissue perfusion indicates body fluid, usually blood, etc. accessing various areas (tissue perfusion) as with cerebral perfusion, perfusing of a kidney for transplantation.

**Perinatal**   *Quick Reference:* Pertaining to birth, being born.
*Advanced Reference:* Indicates the time and process of giving birth.

**Perineal post**   *Quick Reference:* Table attachment involved in patient positioning.
*Advanced Reference:* It is positioned into the peritoneum and acts as a limiting device with a number of orthopaedic table attachments when the patient is positioned for hip/femur surgery. Has the potential for causing injury if care is not applied during positioning, e.g. the genitalia and pudendal nerve.

**Peri-operative**   *Quick Reference:* Indicates the entire operative period.
*Advanced Reference:* Usually indicates the pre-, intra- and post-operative phases of a patient's surgical treatment in one term.

**Peripheral**   *Quick Reference:* (per-if-er-al) Towards the surface of the body.
*Advanced Reference:* Applies to structures close to the surface as opposed to central, as with blood vessels.

**Peristalsis**   *Quick Reference:* Wave of relaxation followed by a wave of contraction, as in the intestinal tract.

*Advanced Reference:* The wave-like motion produced in some body organs to move contents forward. Alternative contraction and relaxation of circular and longitudinal muscles.

**Peritoneum**   *Quick Reference:* Membrane covering the inner walls of the abdominal cavity.

*Advanced Reference:* The peritoneum is a serous membrane and in fact comprises two layers, the *perietal layer* which covers the wall of the cavity and the *visceral layer* which covers the abdominal organs.

**Peroneal**   *Quick Reference:* Relating to the *fibula* and structures on the outer side of the leg.

*Advanced Reference:* Indicates muscles, nerves on the fibular side of the lower leg. The peroneal artery is of significance during positioning patients in the **lithotomy** position, i.e. placing legs on outside or inside of stirrups and causing pressure injury.

**Petri dish**   *Quick Reference:* Glass container used in hospital laboratory.
*Advanced Reference:* A shallow glass dish in which organisms are grown on a culture medium.

**Pexy**   *Quick Reference:* A suffix indicating to fix or suture in place.
*Advanced Reference:* Common example would be orchidopexy, i.e. fixing the testicle into the scrotum.

**Pfannenstiel**   *Quick Reference:* (fan-an-steel) Surgical incision.
*Advanced Reference:* Alternative name for *transverse* incision. Used for such procedures as **Caesarean section** and open *prostatectomy*.

**pH**   *Quick Reference:* Indication of the acid/alkali balance in the body.
*Advanced Reference:* pH measures the number of hydrogen ions in a solution. Acid has a pH below 7, greater than 7 indicates alkaline. Normal pH is in the range of 7.38–7.42.

**Phagocyte**   *Quick Reference:* (fajoo-site) Cells that envelop and digest bacteria.

*Advanced Reference:* Includes the destruction of white blood cells, macrophages, cells and debris. Phagocytes are a vital part of the body's defence system.

**Phalanges**   *Quick Reference:* The bones of the fingers and toes.
*Advanced Reference:* The thumb and big toe have two phalanges, whereas the remaining digits all have three.

**Pharynx**   *Quick Reference:* (far-rinx) Area continuous with the mouth and nasal cavity.

*Advanced Reference:* Muscular back wall of the nose, mouth and throat. Extending from the base of the skull to the entrance of the oesophagus.

The pharynx has three parts or areas; nasopharynx concerned with breathing; the *oropharynx* is a passage for both air and food and the lowest part, the laryngeal pharynx, situated behind the *larynx*, is involved in swallowing.

**Phenol**  *Quick Reference:* (fen-ol) Chemical chiefly used as a disinfectant, e.g. carbolic acid.
*Advanced Reference:* Phenol (carbolic acid) is derived from coal tar and used in many forms and strengths as a disinfectant. Dettol being one well-known preparation. Phenol is also used for nerve block in *chronic* pain and for *sclerotherapy* of haemorrhoids, etc.

**Phimosis**  *Quick Reference:* (fi-mose-is) Tightness of the foreskin so that it cannot be retracted over the head of the penis.
*Advanced Reference:* Common in young children and treated by *circumcision*. Sometimes not actually due to tightness of the foreskin but that the foreskin may still have attachments to underlying tissue until 3–4 years of age.

**Phlebitis**  *Quick Reference:* (flee-bite-is) Inflammation of a vein.
*Advanced Reference:* Generally also associated with blockage of the vessel as in *thrombophlebitis*. May be found at the site of previous IV cannula insertion, due to both inflammation and localised infection.

**Phlebo**  *Quick Reference:* (flee-bo) Prefix indicating vein.
*Advanced Reference:* Phlebo as in phlebotomy, *thrombophlebitis*. Along with veno means pertaining to a vein.

**Phlegm**  *Quick Reference:* (flem) *Mucous.*
*Advanced Reference:* Thick mucous secreted into the nose, throat and bronchial passages.

**Phrenic**  *Quick Reference:* Relating to the diaphragm.
*Advanced Reference:* The phrenic nerve supplies the muscles of the diaphragm. Arises on each side in the neck and passes downwards between the lungs and heart.

**Pia mater**  *Quick Reference:* Innermost of the three membranes that cover the brain and spinal cord.
*Advanced Reference:* A very delicate membrane separated from the arachnoid mater by a space containing the *cerebrospinal fluid* (*CSF*).

**Piggy-back**  *Quick Reference:* Slang term used to indicate one on top of another. A piggy-back ride.
*Advanced Reference:* A piggy-back catheter is one in which an accessory line can be joined to the main lumen. It is common practice to plug an accessory line into the *latex* bung of a *giving-set* via a hypodermic needle.

P

**Pilonidal (sinus)**   *Quick Reference:* Tract containing hair.

*Advanced Reference:* Tract extending to subcuticular level found in the midline of cleft overlying the coccyx and lower sacrum. Treatment is usually surgical excision.

**Pin-index system**   *Quick Reference:* Safety system for connection of medical-gas cylinders.

*Advanced Reference:* An internationally recognised system designed to prevent gas cylinders being connected to the wrong anaesthetic machine yoke. The yoke contains pins which the cylinder head connects to via a set of holes; each individual gas having its unique configuration of pins and holes is identified by numbers, e.g. oxygen = 2 and 5.

**Piped-gas supply**   *Quick Reference:* Form of medical-gas delivery system.

*Advanced Reference:* Indicates the alternative to cylinder supply. Usually involves oxygen and nitrous oxide delivered to theatres, etc. from a cylinder bank (manifold) area or as is usual for $O_2$, from a liquid tank source.

**Piriton**   *Quick Reference:* Proprietary antihistamine, chlorpheniramine.

*Advanced Reference:* Used to treat allergic reactions such as hay fever and *urticaria*.

**Pituitary**   *Quick Reference:* An *endocrine* gland positioned at the base of the brain.

*Advanced Reference:* Also called the hypophysis. Has two lobes, the *anterior* and the *posterior*. The hormones of the anterior lobe are themselves regulated by the *hypothalamus*, which is immediately above the pituitary. Hormones of the pituitary include adrenocorticotrophic hormone (*ACTH*), thyrotrophic, gonadotrophic, growth, lactogenic and melanophore hormones, while the posterior lobe secretes *oxytocin* and antidiuretic hormone (ADH).

**Placebo**   *Quick Reference:* (plas-e-bo) A dummy pill or medicine.

*Advanced Reference:* Any medicine given to placate rather than cure the patient.

**Placenta**   *Quick Reference:* (plas-enter) Organ by which the unborn infant receives nourishment from the mother.

*Advanced Reference:* The placenta is normally firmly attached to the lining of the uterus. Dissolved *oxygen* and nutrients diffuse from the mother's blood to the placenta and *carbon dioxide* and other waste travel in the opposite direction.

**Plasma**   *Quick Reference:* The fluid part of the blood.

*Advanced Reference:* The fluid in which blood cells are suspended or the fluid left after blood has clotted and is called *serum* (i.e. obtained by defibrinating plasma). Total blood volume is comprised of 55% fluid and 45% cells.

**Plasma expander**   *Quick Reference:* IV fluid which increases plasma volume.

*Advanced Reference:* Plasma expanders, e.g. (*colloids*) increase plasma volume via *osmosis*, i.e. drawing fluid from the extracellular and intracellular spaces. *Hypertonic* solutions have similar but shorter-acting effect. Also referred to as *volume expanders*.

**Plasty**   *Quick Reference:* Suffix indicating restorative or reconstructive procedures.

*Advanced Reference:* Most common would be pyeloroplasty and arthroplasty.

**Platelets**   *Quick Reference:* Cells that play a part in blood clotting.

*Advanced Reference: Thrombocytes* or platelets are produced in the bone marrow. An important constituent of blood *coagulation*. They adhere to the walls of injured vessels and help seal them off.

**Plenum**   *Quick Reference:* Operating theatre ventilation system.

*Advanced Reference:* With the plenum system, positive-pressure air, which has been filtered, humidified and warmed (cooled) is fed in at ceiling level and via downward displacement forces air out of lower vents, allowing for approximately 20–30 air changes per hour.

**Pleura**   *Quick Reference:* (plur- ra) The membrane covering the lungs.

*Advanced Reference:* Consists of the *parietal pleura*, which covers the chest wall and the *visceral pleura* which covers the lungs. The space between the two membranes contains a fluid (***surfactant***) which enables the lungs to move freely within the chest.

**Plexus**   *Quick Reference:* A network of structures.

*Advanced Reference:* A network of nerves, blood or lymphatic vessels. An example is the ***brachial plexus*** which is a system of communicating nerve branches at the root of the neck.

**Pneumonectomy**   *Quick Reference:* (nu-mon-ect-omee) Surgical removal of the lung.

*Advanced Reference:* Indicates excision of the whole lung whereas *lobectomy* signifies removal of one lobe of a lung.

**Pneumonia**   *Quick Reference:* (nu-mone-ia) Inflammation of the lungs.

*Advanced Reference:* Due to infection by virus or bacteria. Unlike bronchitis which mostly affects the upper air passages, pneumonia occurs further down the respiratory tract.

**Pneumoperitoneum**   *Quick Reference:* (nu-mo-perit-o-nee-um) Air or gas in the peritoneal cavity.

*Advanced Reference:* In peri-operative terms, refers to insufflation of $CO_2$ prior to laparoscopy.

**Pneumothorax**   *Quick Reference:* (nu-mo-thaw-rax) When air enters the pleural cavity.
*Advanced Reference:* When air gets between the layers of the *pleura* and if the air continues to enter the cavity it could lead to a *tension pneumothorax* which may push the mediastinum over to one side and has the potential to be life threatening.

**Polio (blade)**   *Quick Reference:* Laryngoscope with wide-angled blade popular in obstetric anaesthesia.
*Advanced Reference:* Valuable when patient has large chest/breasts and relatively short neck that will cause intubation difficulties as in late pregnancy. Originally designed for patients treated in iron lung ventilators due to polio.

**Poliomyelitis**   *Quick Reference:* (polio-my-lite-is) Virus infection of the nervous system spread by poor hygiene, pollution of food and water or by droplet infection from the nose.
*Advanced Reference:* Affects the grey matter in front part of the spinal cord affecting the nerve cells responsible for stimulation muscular contraction. If any nerve cells are damaged by the infection, the corresponding muscles can no longer function normally and show signs of wasting.

**Polya**   *Quick Reference:* A type of gastrectomy.
*Advanced Reference:* One form of partial gastrectomy, as alternative to *Billroth*, etc.

**Polycystic**   *Quick Reference:* Characterised by the presence of many cysts.
*Advanced Reference:* Examples are polycystic kidney, liver, ovary.

**Polyethylene**   *Quick Reference:* (poly-eth-i-leen) Strong flexible synthetic resin.
*Advanced Reference:* Produced by the polymerisation of ethylene. Used in the production of many hospital-based products, usually single-use items.

**Polyglactin**   *Quick Reference: Suture* material.
*Advanced Reference:* Synthetic suture material manufactured and distributed as vicryl (coated).

**Polyglycolic acid**   *Quick Reference:* Suture material.
*Advanced Reference:* Synthetic suture manufactured under the name *dexon*.

**Pons**   *Quick Reference:* Prominence on the ventral surface of the brain stem.
*Advanced Reference:* It is situated between the medulla oblongata and the cerebral peduncles of the mid-brain.

**Portal**   *Quick Reference:* Indicates the portal (blood) circulation.

*Advanced Reference:* The portal circulation supplies the liver. Receives all blood from the *alimentary tract*, *pancreas* and *spleen* via the portal vein and its branches which pass through the liver to become the *hepatic* veins.

**Portal hypertension**   *Quick Reference:* A rise (chronic) in the venous pressure in the *portal* circulation.

*Advanced Reference:* The condition is usually caused by obstruction to blood flow through the liver, a major cause being *cirrhosis*.

**Posterior**   *Quick Reference:* Indicates behind.

*Advanced Reference:* Opposite of *anterior*, indicating at the back of or behind, e.g. posterior surface of something.

**Postural drainage**   *Quick Reference:* Drainage of secretions from the lungs.

*Advanced Reference:* Involves the patient laying down, often prone and encouraged to cough up secretions from the lungs. Sometimes accompanied by massage or patting to the sides of the back intended to loosen adherent or thick secretions.

**Potassium**   *Quick Reference:* Most common positively charged particle in the body.

*Advanced Reference:* Symbol K. One of the important electrolytes. Found mainly inside cells and plays a crucial role in nerve conduction and so muscle impulse and contraction. Normal range is 3.5–5.0 mmol/l.

**Pott's fracture**   *Quick Reference:* Generally indicates fracture of the ankle.

*Advanced Reference:* Originally used to indicate a variety of fractures involving the lower ends of the tibia and fibula in the region of the ankle.

**Pouch of Douglas**   *Quick Reference:* Pouch is a pocket-like cavity. Commonly referred to in relation to gynaecology.

*Advanced Reference:* The lowest fold of the peritoneum between the uterus and rectum.

**Povidone**   A polymerised form of vinylpyrrolidone, a white powder soluble in water.

*Advanced Reference:* Used as a dispersing and suspending agent in drugs and other agents. It is combined with *iodine* as a topical antiseptic.

**Practolol**   *Quick Reference:* **Beta-blocker** and **anti-arrhythmic**.

*Advanced Reference:* Used to treat **tachycardia** and irregular heart rhythms. Works by inhibiting the contractile capacity of the heart muscle. Administration is by slow IV injection. Available as Eraldin.

**Precipitation**   *Quick Reference:* (pre-sip-I-tate-on) When a solution forms into solids.

*Advanced Reference:* Applies to drugs, etc. when sometimes mixing two together causes them to solidify or react in a similar way.

**Precursor**   *Quick Reference:* A prognostic characteristic or feature of a patient's health data.

*Advanced Reference:* Examples are X-rays or laboratory findings that are associated with a higher or lower risk of death than average.

**Prednisolone**   *Quick Reference:* Synthetic corticosteroid.

*Advanced Reference:* Used to treat inflammation, especially in rheumatic and allergic conditions.

**Preload**   *Quick Reference:* Strength of ventricular muscle fibres at each diastole.

*Advanced Reference:* It is reflected by ventricular pressure and volume at that part of the cardiac cycle.

**Premedication**   *Quick Reference:* Drug given before surgery.

*Advanced Reference:* Premed or premedication involves drug administration prior to undergoing anaesthetic and surgery. Intended to be a part of the anaesthetic by relieving anxiety, reducing secretions, reducing intra-operative drug doses and diminishing vagal reflexes. Can also involve prophylactic anti-emesis.

**Pressor**   *Quick Reference:* Substance that causes a rise in BP.

*Advanced Reference:* A vasopressor, drug which constricts the blood vessels and raises BP.

**Pressure head**   *Quick Reference:* Highest point of pressure in an irrigation or infusion.

*Advanced Reference:* Refers to the height of an IV infusion or irrigation, and where lies the point from which the highest pressure is exerted, i.e. within the fluid bag, giving-set, etc.

**Priapism**   *Quick Reference:* Persistent erection of the penis.

*Advanced Reference:* The persistent erection is the result of venous thrombosis within the organ. Treatment is usually surgical involving *embolectomy* or venous bypass.

**Prilocaine**   *Quick Reference:* Local anaesthetic (LA).

*Advanced Reference:* Used as an LA for many topical and minor procedures. Available as a cream, solution or for injection. Proprietary versions include *citanest*.

**Primary**   *Quick Reference:* Indicates earliest or first.

*Advanced Reference:* Term used in relation to cancer and its spread. Primary being the initial site and growth of a tumour in relation to secondary, which indicates the further sites the disease could have spread to via *metastasis*.

**Prion**   *Quick Reference:* Protein particle thought to be the cause of various infectious diseases of the nervous system such as *Creutzfeldt–Jakob disease* (CJD).

*Advanced Reference:* The smoke plume from *diathermy* use was thought to be one carrier source of prions involving CJD.

**Procainamide**   *Quick Reference:* A beta-blocker used as an anti-arrhythmic. Available as pronestyl.

*Advanced Reference:* Used to treat heartbeat irregularities especially after heart attack. Owing to its poor absorption properties, has lost popularity as an LA in favour of those that are better absorbed and are longer lasting.

**Procto-colectomy**   *Quick Reference:* Removal of the entire large bowel, rectum and anal canal.

*Advanced Reference:* Performed via a combined abdomino-perineal approach with creation of a permanent *ileostomy* in the right ileac *fossa*.

**Proctoscope**   *Quick Reference:* Instrument for examining the *rectum* and *anal canal*.

*Advanced Reference:* Examination carried out with a *proctoscope*. Related to *sigmoidoscopy* when the rectum and *sigmoid flexure* are examined with a sigmoidoscope.

**Proflavine**   *Quick Reference:* Topical antibacterial cream.

*Advanced Reference:* A formulation of beeswax and liquid paraffin as well as an antibacterial agent, used as a topical application and dressing for minor skin infections, burns and abrasions.

**Prognosis**   *Quick Reference:* To forecast.

*Advanced Reference:* To forecast the probable course and outcome of an illness.

**Prolapse**   *Quick Reference:* The falling forward or downward of an organ.

*Advanced Reference:* A common area for prolapse is the *uterus* which becomes displaced downwards due to weakening of the muscles of the pelvic floor. Causes include childbirth and is treated surgically if necessary. Post-operative problems may involve incontinence.

**Pronation**   *Quick Reference:* To turn the hand palm downwards.

*Advanced Reference:* It is the movement of turning the hand palm downwards or facing backwards. *Prone* position indicates lying face downwards.

**Prone**   *Quick Reference:* Patient lying face down.

*Advanced Reference:* The prone position is when the patient is placed on their front face down. This is most common in spinal surgery, orthopaedics, etc.

**Propagate**   *Quick Reference:* To multiply.

*Advanced Reference:* With regard to animals, plants, etc. To grow (culture) laboratory specimens.

**Prophylaxis**   *Quick Reference:* (pro-fal-axis) Something done to prevent disease.

*Advanced Reference:* Any treatment instituted in order to prevent a disease or condition, e.g. patients are sometimes given prophylactic antibiotics and anti-emetics prior to surgery.

**Propranolol**   *Quick Reference:* **Beta-blocker.**

*Advanced Reference:* Brings about a fall in heart rate and cardiac output combined with a decrease in myocardial oxygen consumption. Used to prevent the reoccurrence of heart attack. Available as Inderal.

**Prostaglandins**   *Quick Reference:* A hormone-type substance produced in numerous parts of the body.

*Advanced Reference:* It is in fact a group of substances which regulate the actions of other hormones and are involved in many body functions, e.g. inflammation, gastric acid secretion, BP adjustment, clotting, renal elimination and immunity. They increase the contraction of smooth muscle, particularly in the uterus and are used to induce abortion. May also be used to induce labour. Available as synthetic versions.

**Prostate**   *Quick Reference:* Gland surrounding the neck of the bladder and beginning of the urethra in men.

*Advanced Reference:* The prostate produces a fluid which forms part of the *semen*. In later life it is liable to benign enlargement which may obstruct urine flow. If warranted, surgery is required to remove it or reduce the size of the gland.

**Prosthesis**   *Quick Reference:* Artificial substitute for a body part.

*Advanced Reference:* Technically involves false teeth, glass eye, false leg, etc. but with reference to theatres usually indicates, e.g. a hip, knee replacement, etc.

**Protamine**   *Quick Reference:* An *antidote* for heparin.

*Advanced reference:* An **antagonist** of the *anticoagulant* heparin, the action of which normally lasts approximately 4–6 h but this time can be speeded up by the administration of protamine. Used regularly during *cardiopulmonary bypass*, renal dialysis.

**Protocol**   *Quick Reference:* A written plan.

*Advanced Reference:* A plan which specifies the procedures to be followed, e.g. an examination, research or when providing care.

**Proximal**   *Quick Reference:* Nearest to the centre of the body.

*Advanced Reference:* Describes anything which is nearer to a given point of reference. In anatomy, the centre point of the body is taken as the reference point. The opposite being *distal*.

**Pseudomonas**   *Quick Reference:* (sude-a-moan-us) Gram-negative bacilli.
 *Advanced Reference:* One type, *Pseudomonas aeruginosa*, infects wounds, burns, etc. and is found in water traps, humidifiers, etc.

**PTFE**   *Quick Reference:* Teflon (polytetrafluoroethylene).
 *Advanced Reference:* Substance with non-stick properties developed via space race (National Aeronautics and Space Administration, NASA). IV cannulae can be either coated or made from Teflon. This property helps reduce thrombus formation and can help increase flow rate.

**Pudendal**   *Quick Reference:* Nerve that supplies the *perineum, vulva* and lower *vagina*.
 *Advanced Reference:* Nerve that can be damaged by a peroneal post when patient is positioned for hip/femur surgery on orthopaedic table, etc. Pudendal nerve block, used in obstetrics for vaginal/forceps delivery, *episiotomy*, etc.

**Pulseless electrical activity**   *Quick Reference:* Condition related to advanced cardiac life support (ACLS).
 *Advanced Reference:* Condition where there is an absence of a pulse in conjunction with a relatively normal looking ECG. Common causes are *hypovolaemia, hypoxia, hypothermia*, etc.

**Purse-string**   *Quick Reference:* Type of *suture* used to close an opening.
 *Advanced Reference:* A continuous circular suture placed around an opening and can cause it to close. As with *appendix* removal, or the urinary bladder when inserting a drainage tube.

**Pus**   *Quick Reference:* Yellowish fluid that is a by-product of inflammation/infection.
 *Advanced Reference:* Tissue fluid containing dead white cells, bacteria and broken-down tissues. Has a distinctive smell but this is dependent on the type of bacteria involved.

**Putrefaction**   *Quick Reference:* The breaking down of tissue by bacteria.
 *Advanced Reference:* Refers to the changes that take place in bodies of animals and plants after death. Almost entirely due to bacterial action which reduces living matter to carbonic acid gas, ammonia, etc. Usually accompanied by offensive odour due to gases produced.

**Putti-Platt operation**   *Quick Reference:* Orthopaedic procedure for shoulder dislocation.
 *Advanced Reference:* The procedure is performed to prevent recurrent dislocation of the shoulder.

**P-wave**   *Quick Reference:* Component of electrocardiographical (ECG) trace.
 *Advanced Reference:* The first wave or deflection on the ECG trace, it indicates contraction of the atria.

**Pyelogram**   *Quick Reference:* Radiological examination of the renal pelvis.
*Advanced Reference:* Radio-opaque dye is injected IV and after approximately 10 min X-rays are taken to outline the area. Retrograde pyelogram involves inserting dye into the renal pelvis using a ***cystoscope*** and *ureteric* catheter.

**Pylorus**   *Quick Reference:* Aperture in the stomach through which food passes into the duodenum.
*Advanced Reference:* The pylorus is surrounded by a circular muscle (*pyloric sphincter*) which controls opening and closing of the aperture.

**Pyrexia**   *Quick Reference:* Fever.
*Advanced Reference:* Condition in which the body temperature is above normal.

**Pyrogen**   *Quick Reference:* Any substance which produces a fever.
*Advanced Reference:* Any substance capable of producing pyrexia or the possibility of a ***pathogenic*** reaction. Pyrogens are produced by bacteria during the manufacture and storage of IV fluids and although the bacteria are killed during the sterilisation process, their pyrogenic protein particles are left behind and can lead to reactions.

**Pyuria**   *Quick Reference:* Pus in the urine.
*Advanced Reference:* Due to inflammation/infection in the urinary tract.

**QRS-complex** *Quick Reference:* Represents ventricular depolarisation.

*Advanced Reference:* Normal duration is approximately 0.12 s. The Q-wave is the initial downward deflection of the QRS-complex. The QT-interval represents the duration of ventricular systole.

**Quack** *Quick Reference:* A charlatan, fraud.

*Advanced Reference:* Term applied to someone (impersonating another or pretending to be what they are not (professionally), commonly a medical doctor).

**Quadrants** *Quick Reference:* Areas, regions and quarters.

*Advanced Reference:* The abdominal and pelvic areas of the trunk are divided into quadrants, i.e. right upper and lower quadrants and left upper and lower quadrants.

**Quadriceps** *Quick Reference:* The large muscle covering the front of the thigh.

*Advanced Reference:* The main combination of four muscles within the lower limbs that give structure and mobility to extension and straightening of the knee.

**Quadriplegia** *Quick Reference:* Paralysis of all four limbs.

*Advanced Reference:* Also termed *tetraplegia*.

**Qualitative** *Quick Reference:* Pertaining to quality.

*Advanced Reference:* The value or nature of something. Determines the presence or absence of a substance.

**Quality assurance** *Quick Reference:* Also known as quality management. An aspect of general and hospital management. Indicates a standard or level of excellence.

*Advanced Reference:* A management system that assures quality with the work for which one is responsible.

**Quantiflex** *Quick Reference:* Type of anaesthetic machine.

*Advanced Reference:* This machine is common in dental anaesthesia. It has a number of specific features, i.e. separated flowmetres, one common control knob that adjusts total gas flow (oxygen and nitrous), and most notably that the design prevents delivery of hypoxic mixtures with the capacity to deliver no lower than 30% oxygen.

**Quantitative**   *Quick Reference:* Capable of being measured.
*Advanced Reference:* Quantitative analysis is the determination of the amounts of constituents in a sample.

**Quart**   *Quick Reference:* Unit of fluid volume.
*Advanced Reference:* Fluid measure equivalent to one-quarter of a gallon, or two pints, 32 fluid ounces, 946.24 ml.

**Quinidine**   *Quick Reference:* A drug obtained from the cinchona tree called delanide.
*Advanced Reference:* Used in the treatment of irregular heart action (cardiac arrhythmias), more specifically, ventricular extrasystoles and ventricular tachycardia.

**Quinine**   *Quick Reference:* Alkaloid made from the bark of the cinchona tree.
*Advanced Reference:* Used as a remedy in malaria and can be given orally or intravenously (IV).

**Quinsy**   *Quick Reference:* Abscess surrounding the tonsil.
*Advanced Reference:* Peritonsillar abscess, where infection has occurred in the surrounding tissue of the tonsil area. Characterised by symptoms of sore throat, fever and difficulty swallowing. Treated initially with antibiotics; however, extreme cases will require surgical intervention.

**Quintuplet**   *Quick Reference:* Five-fold.
*Advanced Reference:* Five offspring born at the same *gestation* period during a single pregnancy.

**Quotient**   *Quick Reference:* Result from dividing one quantity by another.
*Advanced Reference:* The respiratory quotient is the ratio between the carbon dioxide expired and the oxygen inspired during a specified time.

**R**

**Radiation** *Quick Reference:* Energy in the form of electromagnetic waves.
  *Advanced Reference:* May be *ionising* or *non-ionising.* Examples are gamma rays, X-rays, infrared, ultraviolet, microwaves.

**Radical** *Quick Reference:* Taking an extensive clearing. Radical surgery is extensive enough to be curative rather than *palliative.*
  *Advanced Reference:* Often referred to as radical-wide excision. This would imply that extra tissue is to be removed in order to ensure all affected or diseased tissues are removed.

**Radioactive** *Quick Reference:* A chemical substance giving off radiation.
  *Advanced Reference:* Atoms that have the same number of protons and different numbers of neutrons are commonly referred to as *isotopes.* A number of isotopes pose threats to human life mainly due to their unstable nature, thus caused by a breakdown in their nuclei.

**Radiographer** *Quick Reference:* (raid-eog-rafer) X-ray technician.
  *Advanced Reference:* The radiographer is responsible for the production of films and images for the radiologist to diagnose.

**Radiology** *Quick Reference:* Medical speciality concerned with the use of electromagnetic radiation.
  *Advanced Reference:* Radiologists can be either diagnostic or therapeutic. Besides the diagnosis of X-rays, computerised tomography (CT) and magnetic resonance imaging (MRI) scans, the former are becoming increasingly involved in invasive treatment of many conditions that were once treated solely with open surgery. Therapeutic radiologists are primarily concerned with utilising radioactive materials to treat disease, e.g. cancers.

**Radio-opaque** *Quick Reference:* Substance capable of obstructing X-rays.
  *Advanced Reference:* Also referred to as contrast medium, used in X-ray procedures as a dye to produce an outline or image of an area, e.g. blood vessel, biliary tree.

**Radiotherapy** *Quick Reference:* Treatment of disease by radioactive substances.

*Advanced Reference:* This could be achieved through the use of X-rays to identify the nature of a fracture or underlying disease in any area of the patient's anatomy. Other more direct uses of radioactive substances in radiotherapy could be the insertion of the material within the patient close to the tumour. Most common radioactive substance used in radiotherapy are sealed capsules of cobalt 60.

**Radium**   *Quick Reference:* Radioactive element.
*Advanced Reference:* Radioactive isotopes are utilised in radiotherapy for destroying cancer cells.

**Radius**   *Quick Reference:* Bone of the forearm.
*Advanced Reference:* The outer bone of the lower arm is smaller than the *ulna* which it accompanies.

**Rales**   *Quick Reference:* (rails) Abnormal sounds heard via a stethoscope when examining the chest.
*Advanced Reference:* Usually due to disease of the lungs involving fluid, etc. in the air passages. The sound is produced by air passing over or through dry or wet secretions.

**Ramsted's procedure**   *Quick Reference:* Operation performed for stricture of the pylorus.
*Advanced Reference:* Named after the German surgeon W.C Ramstedt. Performed for congenital stricture or stenosis of the pylorus. The condition is usually detected in a newborn having difficulty retaining milk. Projectile vomiting is associated with this condition. A longitudinal incision is made into the pylorus and then resutured transversely creating a wider inner opening between the pylorus and the duodenum. Otherwise known as a *pyloroplasty*.

**Ranitidine**   *Quick Reference:* Antacid or $H_2$ receptor antagonist.
*Advanced Reference:* Rantidine is used to reduce gastric acid output by blocking the function of the $H_2$ receptors. Indications for use are reflux within the oesophagus and gastric ulcers.

**Ranula**   *Quick Reference:* A retention cyst found under the tongue on either side of the frenum.
*Advanced Reference:* Caused by the sublingual duct or mucous glands becoming obstructed.

**Rash**   *Quick Reference:* Temporary eruption or discolouration of the skin.
*Advanced Reference:* Often associated with allergy, infection, fever, reaction, etc.

**Ratchet**   *Quick Reference:* A toothed bar with an interlocking device.
*Advanced Reference:* The toothed bar of a ratchet can be found on one side of the handles of artery forceps. The other side contains the corresponding

tooth that locks into place when applied. Artery forceps are stored and passed to the surgeon on the first ratchet. This allows maximum dexterity for the surgeon when applying an artery forceps during an emergency bleeding situation. The ratchet gives adequate strength to the artery forceps to remain *in situ*. A number of additional instruments utilise ratchets, i.e. mouth gags.

**Raynaud's disease** *Quick Reference:* (ray-nards) Condition in which the fingers and toes become cold and white or blue when exposed to cold.

*Advanced Reference:* Occurs usually in young women. Produces numbness, tingling and can be painful. Also signified by becoming red when warmed and again can produce tingling and pain. The cause is spasm of the arterioles supplying the digits. There is no specific treatment although drugs and surgery are sometimes used. Surgery involves the interruption of the sympathetic nerves (*sympathectomy*).

**Raytec** *Quick Reference:* Often referred to as Raytec swabs.

*Advanced Reference:* The Raytec referred to within surgical swabs is the actual translucent lining through the middle of the swab. Its purpose is to highlight the swab on X-ray, should a swab be mislaid during a surgical procedure. Other similar materials are used in endotracheal (ET) tubes, ureteric stents, catheters. Essentially, it is a protective measure to ensure nothing is left inside the patient after procedures.

**RDS** *Quick Reference:* Respiratory distress syndrome.

*Advanced Reference:* Involves the development of dyspnoea soon after birth in premature babies and is characterised by chest retraction accompanied by cyanosis and grunting on expiration.

**Reamer** *Quick Reference:* Surgical instrument used in orthopaedics and dentistry.

*Advanced Reference:* Used for enlarging root canals in dentistry and clearing out the shaft of bones for prosthesis insertion, i.e. shaft of femur for hip replacement.

**Receiver** *Quick Reference:* A kidney-shaped dish.

*Advanced Reference:* A receiver is used during surgery to contain any patient fluids, dissected body tissue, etc. It is also a best practice to pass the surgical blade between the scrub practitioner and the surgeon in a receiver in an attempt to reduce injury to either professional. Generally speaking, receivers/kidney dishes can be used as a general-purpose container whether sterile or non-sterile.

**Receptor** *Quick Reference:* Nerve ending adapted to a particular kind of sensation or a chemical component of a living cell.

*Advanced Reference:* Receptors receive stimuli in order to bring about a reaction or change.

**Recipient**   *Quick Reference:* One who receives.

*Advanced Reference:* One who receives blood from another. The universal recipient is someone who can receive blood from all groups of *donors.* Also, a recipient receiving a donated organ for **transplantation.**

**Recovery**   *Quick Reference:* Refers to the recovery area of theatre suits.

*Advanced Reference:* Now more regularly being referred to as post-anaesthetic care unit (PACU) and in some centres also functions as a high-dependency unit (HDU).

**Rectocele**   *Quick Reference:* (rec-toe-seal) Prolapse of the **rectum.**

*Advanced Reference:* Occurs commonly in women following childbirth and due to overstretching of the vaginal wall.

**Rectum**   *Quick Reference:* Last section of the large intestines.

*Advanced Reference:* The last few inches of the intestine, terminating in the anal canal, sigmoid flexure to anus.

**Rectus sheath**   *Quick Reference:* A covering over the rectus abdominis muscle.

*Advanced Reference:* It is a thick sheath of connective tissue which covers the *rectus abdominis* muscle.

**Recumbent**   *Quick Reference:* Lying down, reclining.

*Advanced Reference:* A recumbent position, sometimes used to describe or infer supine.

**Recurrent**   *Quick Reference:* To recur. Happening time after time. Turning back so as to renew direction.

*Advanced Reference:* An example in anatomy is the recurrent laryngeal nerve where one branch loops under the subclavian artery on the right side and under the arch of the aorta on the left, then returns upward to the larynx to supply all the muscles of the thyroid, except the cricothyroid.

**Redivac**   *Quick Reference:* Pre-vacuumed surgical drain.

*Advanced Reference:* Pre-vacuumed sterile portable, self-contained closed wound suction unit. A Redivac drain is used intra-operatively and gives a more accurate blood loss post-surgery.

**Reducing valve**   *Quick Reference:* Pressure-regulating valve.

*Advanced Reference:* Device for reducing high-pressure delivery of gases to anaesthetic machines and maintaining the reduced pressure at a manageable level.

**Reduction**   *Quick Reference:* Correction of or decrease in size.

*Advanced Reference:* (i) The correction of a fracture or dislocation of a bone. (ii) The measures taken to reduce a hernia by surgical operation to ensure that the abdominal organs remain within the cavity while the weak muscle lining is repaired. (iii) Refers to a breast reduction, the cosmetic surgery to make the breast size smaller.

**Re-fashioning**  *Quick Reference:* Surgical re-suturing or re-anchoring of a structure.

*Advanced Reference:* Essentially this is the re-suturing of a structure previously made during surgery. Re-fashioning of a colostomy, would be to re-site or correct the *stoma* on the skin surface.

**Reflex**  *Quick Reference:* Involuntary response to a stimulus.

*Advanced Reference:* This is the automatic reaction by the body to a stimulus, determined by impulses in nerves, e.g. a knee-jerk.

**Reflux**  *Quick Reference:* Backward flow.

*Advanced Reference:* Term used to indicate *regurgitation* as with gastro-oesophageal reflux, etc. due to *hiatus hernia*.

**Refraction**  *Quick Reference:* The deviation of light rays from a straight pathway.

*Advanced Reference:* In medicine, refraction refers to the focusing mechanism of the eye.

**Regurgitation**  *Quick Reference:* The back flow of gastric contents into the mouth.

*Advanced Reference:* Regurgitation is a passive act while vomiting is active and requires muscle tone. Therefore, patients administered a muscle relaxant for general anaesthetic (GA) regurgitate. If this occurs can be aspirated into the lungs and lead to *Mendelson's syndrome*.

**Rejection**  *Quick Reference:* Refers to the rejection of transplanted organs.

*Advanced Reference:* Involves the host forming antibodies against the transplanted tissue, leading to eventual rejection.

**Relative humidity**  *Quick Reference:* This is the ratio of the mass of water vapour in a given volume of the air to the mass.

*Advanced Reference:* Relative humidity is the absolute humidity divided by the amount present when the gas(air) is fully saturated at the same temperature and pressure. Applicable to theatre environment where it should be approximately 50% to 55% and measured with a *hygrometer*.

**Relaxant**  *Quick Reference:* Refers to muscle-relaxant drugs. To paralyse the patient.

*Advanced Reference:* Used to provide loss of muscle tone for surgery and intubation. Includes both *depolarising* and *non-depolarising* types.

**Religion and culture**  *Quick Reference:* Refers to the varied treatment requirements of diverse groups.

*Advanced Reference:* Although staff have always been aware of the specific needs in relation to culture and religion (Jehovah's Witnesses, etc.), the issue has gained prominence in recent years and at all stages staff must be aware of any aspects of treatment that could be contra to beliefs. Patients should be consulted regarding any areas of concern and all staff should receive appropriate training so to avoid potential infringement and possible discrimination.

**Remifentanil**   *Quick Reference:* Opioid analgesic.

*Advanced Reference:* Short-acting opioid, popularly used as an infusion during anaesthesia.

**Remission**   *Quick Reference:* The active process of surrendering, resigning or retreating.

*Advanced Reference:* A temporary and incomplete subsidence of the active source of pain, infection or more serious illness. Often referred to in the context that a patient's cancer has gone into remission. This would indicate that the symptoms have eased or disease progress slowed or halted.

**Renal**   *Quick Reference:* Relating to the kidney.

*Advanced Reference:* Located or affecting the region of the kidney.

**Renal failure**   *Quick Reference:* Inability of the kidney to carry out its normal functions.

*Advanced Reference:* May be acute or chronic. Acute renal failure (ARF) may be due to trauma and shock, when a lengthy drop in blood pressure (BP) may be the cause and function may/should return after a period of perfusion or dialysis. Chronic renal failure (CRF) failure can be due to a number of disease processes and involves long-term dialysis and eventual transplantation.

**Rendell-Baker**   *Quick Reference:* Commonly refers to a design of paediatric face mask.

*Advanced Reference:* Designed to minimise dead space by being anatomically moulded to fit the face.

**Renin**   *Quick Reference:* Hormone formed by the kidneys.

*Advanced Reference:* Concerned with the regulation of BP. Released into the bloodstream by the renal arterioles when kidneys are damaged or ischaemic and causes vasoconstriction and so a rise in BP.

**Rennin**   *Quick Reference:* An enzyme present in gastric juice.

*Advanced Reference:* Responsible for clotting the protein casein, as the first step in the digestion of milk.

**Resection**   *Quick Reference:* The surgical removal of an organ or structure.

*Advanced Reference:* Used commonly to indicate general cutting and removal during surgery.

**Resectoscope**   *Quick Reference:* Surgical instrument used in urology.
*Advanced Reference:* A cutting attachment used in conjunction with a telescope passed back down the urethra to reduce the size of the prostate by cutting and shaving (*TURP*).

**Reservoir bag**   *Quick Reference:* Bag incorporated into anaesthetic-breathing systems.
*Advanced Reference:* Its function is to store gases and provide them for continued ventilation. Can also be an indicator of breathing pattern and efficiency during spontaneous respiration.

**Residual/residue**   *Quick Reference:* Relating to, or being something that remains.
*Advanced Reference:* Can refer to the residual volume in the lungs after a maximum expiration. Residue left in the bladder following urination.

**Resistance**   *Quick Reference:* Power or capacity to resist.
*Advanced Reference:* Examples could be electrical resistance or resistance in breathing systems, especially in relation to paediatrics.

**Respirometer**   *Quick Reference:* Device for measuring expiratory gas volumes.
*Advanced Reference:* Found in different designs (electronic and mechanical) in anaesthetic apparatus (*Wright's*) as well as for testing lung capacity and capability.

**Resusci-Annie**   *Quick Reference:* A *cardiopulmonary* resuscitation (CPR) training manikin.
*Advanced Reference:* An education tool used for teaching CPR. Various models are available but primarily they respond to attempts of rescue breathing and external cardiac massage. Available in child and adult sizes.

**Resuscitaire**   *Quick Reference:* (re-sus-sit-air) A specially designed resuscitation trolley for newborn.
*Advanced Reference:* Resuscitaires are a moveable trolley that has a sloping bed (head down) for the newborn. This device is used to resuscitate and/or monitor the newborn for normal respiration, cardiac function and adequate oxygenation. The resuscitaire has suction, oxygen delivery, overhead heating lamp and accessories required immediately following delivery.

**Resuscitation**   *Quick Reference:* (re-sus-sit-a-shon) To revive, try to bring back to normal.
*Advanced Reference:* Term used to indicate the process of reviving someone (apparently dead or dying), using CPR techniques. However, is used to cover the treatment of shock and stabilise patients with intravenous (IV) fluids, medication, oxygen, etc.

**Retching**   *Quick Reference:* Involuntary spasm related to vomiting.

*Advanced Reference:* Although used in relation to vomiting, actually indicates ineffectual effort and being non-productive.

**Retention**   *Quick Reference:* The act of keeping back.

*Advanced Reference:* A common example would be urinary retention which involves the inability to void urine from the bladder, usually due to obstruction.

**Retina**   *Quick Reference:* The innermost layer of the eye ball involved in the receiving of images.

*Advanced Reference:* Light-sensitive membrane lining the back of the eye consisting of several layers of nerve cells and fibres containing the rods and cones. The images reach the brain by way of the optic nerve.

**Retractors**   *Quick Reference:* An instrument used during surgery.

*Advanced Reference:* A retractor is used to hold open a wound or cavity or pull tissue aside to give the surgeon room to work and provide a better view. They come in many shapes and sizes depending on the area of the body they are designed for. Some of the most common being Devers, Czerny, Volkman, double or single Skin Hooks, Walton's malleable retractor, West Mastoid, Traverse, Balfour and Roux, etc.

**Retrograde**   *Quick Reference:* Going against the normal direction. The prefix retro indicates going backwards.

*Advanced Reference:* Occurring or performed in a direction opposite to the usual direction of conduction or flow. Retrograde priming is carried out when preparing IV infusions, retrograde *prostatectomy* is another term for *TURP*, i.e. going back down the urethra. A retropubic prostatectomy is an open technique involving going behind the pubic bone to access the prostate for removal.

**Retroversion**   *Quick Reference:* Backward displacement of an organ.

*Advanced Reference:* Pertaining to the uterus. A normal uterus slopes downwards and backwards and a retroverted uterus may lie vertically or slope downwards and forwards.

**Retrovirus**   *Quick Reference:* A group of viruses.

*Advanced Reference:* These viruses infect and destroy helper T-cells of the immune system. Human immunodeficiency virus (HIV), the virus responsible for acquired human immunodeficiency syndrome (AIDS), is a member of this group.

**Rhesus factor**   *Quick Reference:* (re-sus) (Rh factor) Rhesus blood group system.

*Advanced Reference:* A group of antigens that may or may not be present on the surface of the red blood cells. People with this factor are

Rh-positive and those who lack the factor are Rh-negative. Incompatibility between the two is a cause of transfusion reactions and of haemolytic disease of the newborn.

**Rheumatoid** *Quick Reference:* (ru-mat-oid) Disorders effected by inflammation and degeneration.

*Advanced Reference:* Relates to disorders such as arthritis, and indicates the added effects to the condition.

**Rhinoplasty** *Quick Reference:* Rhino meaning nose; corrective nasal surgery.

*Advanced Reference:* Surgical procedure performed to alter the shape and size of the nose usually for cosmetic reasons.

**Rhys-Davis exanguinator** *Quick Reference:* A limb exanguinator used prior to the application of a tourniquet in orthopaedic surgery.

*Advanced Reference:* A black rubber (sausage) device that has a central hole through which a patient's arm or leg can be inserted. The rolling effect over the limb coupled with the internal pressure of the device squeezes blood out of the veins. Once placed up to the level of the tourniquet, which is then inflated, this stops arterial flow into the limb and so creating a bloodless field.

**Rib** *Quick Reference:* A curved bone that forms part of the thoracic cage.

*Advanced Reference:* There are 12 pairs of ribs within the thoracic cage of the human body. Each rib is flat and curved and joined at the spinal vertebrae by cartilage. The top seven pairs of ribs are directly connected to the sternum while the remaining five pairs are classified as *false ribs* connected to each other by cartilage. The last two pairs of the false ribs are often referred to as floating ribs because they are attached to the vertebrae at the back but are not connected at the front. Ribs are useful landmarks for identifying key insertion points for intercostal chest drains, subclavian vein cannulae, etc.

**RIDDOR** *Quick Reference:* Reporting of injuries, diseases and dangerous occurrences.

*Advanced Reference:* Part of the *Health and Safety Regulations* for ensuring the safety of all within the organisational setting. The report details the systematic process for reporting and recording relevant details of accidents, etc. It also gives a time frame for when the reports are to be completed and forwarded to the Health and Safety Executive/Commission for further investigation.

**Rigor** *Quick Reference:* Intense shivering.

*Advanced Reference:* Involves shivering and a sensation of coldness accompanied by a rise in temperature. Often indicates fever in combination with sweating. *Rigor mortis* is the stiffening of the body that occurs within approximately 8 hours of death and is due to changes in muscle tissue.

**Ring block**  *Quick Reference:* Subcuticular infiltration of local anaesthetic (LA).

*Advanced Reference:* Used to anaesthetise extremities such as fingers and toes. Involves infiltrating LA subcuticularly around the full circumference of the extremity proximal to the site. Useful for emergency situations prior to toilet and suturing.

**Ringers lactate**  *Quick Reference:* IV maintenance and replacement solution.

*Advanced Reference:* IV fluid consisting mainly of normal saline with small amounts of calcium and potassium.

**Risk management**  *Quick Reference:* Process initially involved with managing health and safety within a department.

*Advanced Reference:* Involves highlighting an activity and assessing the risks in comparison to need and then making changes and/or substitutions.

**Robert-Shaw tube**  *Quick Reference:* A double-lumen ET tube with an angled end to right or left.

*Advanced Reference:* Used and designed for *one-lung anaesthesia.* Comes in right and left design and varying sizes, with *non-disposable* being small, medium and large and the *disposable* type mostly supplied in French gauge. Has two channels and is used with either a single- or double-catheter mount connection to facilitate one- or two-lung ventilation. Both have a tracheal and bronchial cuff. The right-sided version has an eye to facilitate right upper lobe ventilation.

**Robinul**  *Quick Reference:* A proprietary **anticholinergic** drug.

*Advanced Reference:* It is a preparation of glycopyrronium bromide (*glycopyrrolate*) used in combination with **neostigmine** for reversal of *non-depolarising* muscle relaxants.

**Rocuronium**  *Quick Reference: Non-depolorising* muscle relaxant.

*Advanced Reference:* Neuromuscular-blocking drug that has a fast onset of action, excreted in the kidneys and chemically similar to *vecuronium.*

**Rodent ulcer**  *Quick Reference:* A malignant **tumour** of the skin.

*Advanced Reference:* Arises from the basal cells and is usually found on the face, particularly in those who have been exposed to the sun. Has the appearance of a raised ulcer that will not heal. Does not give rise to secondary growths in other parts of the body but if left it is capable of spreading into the bone beneath the skin.

**Rogitine**  *Quick Reference:* Proprietary **antihypertensive.**

*Advanced Reference:* An alpha-blocker used to treat hypertension and heart failure, i.e. phentolamine.

**Roller-ball**  *Quick Reference:* A control clamp on an IV administration set.

*Advanced Reference:* The roller-ball is a controlling clamp fitted to an IV infusion set downstream of the chambers, designed to control the flow of fluid through the giving-set.

**Ronguer** *Quick Reference:* (ron-jure) A surgical instrument used for nibbling bone.

*Advanced Reference:* Derived from the French word meaning to nibble. Usually used to bite off (nibble) small pieces of bone in orthopaedics and neurosurgery.

**Ropivacaine** *Quick Reference:* LA drug.

*Advanced Reference:* Similar to *bupivacaine*, but less cardiotoxic.

**Rotameter** *Quick Reference:* Trade name of a type of *flowmeter*.

*Advanced Reference:* A type of flowmeter used in anaesthetic machines. It consists of a glass-tapered tube (wider at the top) mounted vertically within which a rotating bobbin is free to move up the tube, indicating flow and volume delivered. The tapered shape creates an annular orifice between the bobbin and the walls of the tubing and this orifice increases in size as the bobbin moves up the tube, controlled by the needle valve.

**Rotary clamp** *Quick Reference:* Operating table fixation device.

*Advanced Reference:* Type of fixation clamp used to attach table fittings such as *Carter Braine* arm rests, back rests, etc. Its design (rotary) allows for adjustment not possible with fixed clamps, e.g. creating low *lithotomy*, etc. but extra vigilance is required as the nature of the clamp can lead to a less-stable fixation.

**Round-bodied needles** *Quick Reference:* Refers to a suture needle which has a rounded shaft but a sharp tapered point for passing through delicate tissues.

*Advanced Reference:* Round-bodied needles are used for approximation of soft tissues and are designed to separate body tissues rather than cut them. Examples would be when suturing bowel tissues.

**Roux-en-Y** *Quick Reference:* (ru-en-why) A type of anastomosis.

*Advanced Reference:* An anastomosis of the small intestine in the shape of the letter 'Y'. The proximal end of the divided intestine is anastamosed end to side to the distal loop and a part of the distal loop is anastomosed to another part of the digestive tract, e.g. the *oesophagus*.

**Rowbotham connector** *Quick Reference:* (row-bottom) A metal connector inserted into a red rubber ET tube.

*Advanced Reference:* It is of a right-angled design and was used in both oral and nasal ET tubes. Now superseded by pre-formed tubes.

**RTA** *Quick Reference:* Road traffic accident.

*Advanced Reference:* A term still in use throughout critical care areas of hospitals but gradually being replaced with the motor vehicle collision (MVC).

**Rubber shod** *Quick Reference:* A protective cover placed over the ends of fine artery forceps, e.g. halsteads.

*Advanced Reference:* May be made of rubber or a fine size 10G catheter. When placed over the ends of the artery forceps it makes the forceps less traumatic. Therefore, can then be use to hold fine sutures, e.g. 7/0, 8/0, etc.

**Ruben valve**   *Quick Reference:* A non-rebreathing valve.

*Advanced Reference:* A one-way valve, similar in design and function to the Ambu valve. Allows for a constant flow of fresh gas, as there is no mixing of fresh and expired gases. Seldom used in anaesthetics but still found in resuscitation-type circuits, i.e. bag-valve-mask (*BVM*).

**Rule of Nines**   *Quick Reference:* Assessment measuring system used in relation to patients with burns.

*Advanced Reference:* Used for external burns to make an estimate of the percentage area burned. For an adult each of the following areas affected is taken as 9% of the total body area: front of thorax, back of thorax, front of abdomen, back of abdomen, each arm, front of each leg, back of each leg, head plus neck. The area of the perineum is about 1%. In children, the head is assessed as 15–20% due to being proportionately much greater. Another useful measure is the front of the patient's hand, which represents about 1% of the surface area.

**Ryles tube**   *Quick Reference:* A plastic-weighted tube inserted into the gastric system through the nasopharyngeal route.

*Advanced Reference:* Also termed nasogastric tube. Available in varying sizes and contains a radio-opaque line and metal ball in the tip for weighting. Used during gastric, hepatic and bowel surgery to allow escape of gas and gastric fluid. In theatres, they are often stored in the fridge to give a degree of rigidity to help insertion, which is usually carried out once the patient is anaesthetised.

# S

**Sacrum** *Quick Reference:* (say-crumb) Bone at the base of the spinal column.
*Advanced Reference:* Triangular bone formed by the fusion of five *vertebrae*. It forms above with the lumbar vertebrae and below with the coccyx.

**Sagital** *Quick Reference:* An imaginary line extending from front to back.
*Advanced Reference:* In the midline of the body, dividing right and left parts.

**Saliva** *Quick Reference:* Commonly referred to as spittle.
*Advanced Reference:* Secretion of the salivary glands which contains water, mucous, ptyalin and starts the process of digestion.

**Salmonella** *Quick Reference:* The main cause of food poisoning.
*Advanced Reference:* Genus of Gram-negative bacteria. Parasites of the gastrointestinal tract responsible for common types of food poisoning as well as typhoid and paratyphoid fevers.

**Saphenous** *Quick Reference:* (saf-een-us) Refers to veins in the lower leg.
*Advanced Reference:* The long saphenous vein runs up the inside of the leg from the ankle to the groin and the short saphenous from the outside of the ankle to the back of the knee. The long saphenous is the longest vein in the body. Often used in vascular and cardiac surgery as a source for a graft.

**Sarcoma** *Quick Reference:* A tumour of connective tissue often highly malignant.
*Advanced Reference:* May occur in any part of the body and tends to grow rapidly and metastasises early to distant sites.

**Savlodil** *Quick Reference:* An antiseptic. Savlon.
*Advanced Reference:* Produced in the form of sterile sachets and is a compound preparation of the disinfectants *chlorhexidine* gluconate and *cetrimide*.

**Scavenging system** *Quick Reference:* Method of removing waste gases in theatres.

*Advanced Reference:* More specifically, removes the waste gases from the expiratory ports of anaesthetic-breathing systems. Can be passive or active. Passive systems are rarely used now and involve directing the gases to a carbon-filled container (*Cardiff Aldasorber*), which absorbs some vapours or simply involve leading gases away via a length of tubing to an exterior area. Active systems utilise low vacuum as an aid to extraction.

**Schimmelbusch mask**   *Quick Reference:* (shim-em-bush) Early design of anaesthetic mask for delivering anaesthetic volatile agents.

*Advanced Reference:* Although referred to as a mask, is also classified as a vaporiser. Was in fact a wire-mask-shaped frame which fitted over the patient's mouth and nose then covered with gauze. The anaesthetic was then sprinkled onto the gauze which became impregnated and consequently the patient inhaled the vapours. Concentration was determined simply by the amount of liquid sprinkled on the gauze.

**Schraeder**   *Quick Reference:* (shrader) Design of anaesthetic gas pipeline fitting/valve.

*Advanced Reference:* Classed as a valve or simply fitting, refers to the couplings for oxygen, nitrous oxide, air and suction, which are usually wall-mounted or hang from the theatre ceiling. The valve ensures that the gas is shut off when no probe is in place and are colour coded and unique to each gas.

**Scirrhous**   *Quick Reference:* (skir-us) A type of cancer.

*Advanced Reference:* Pertaining to a hard tumour. Or scirrhus, a growth of connective tissue, such as a hard carcinoma of the breast.

**Scissors**   *Quick Reference:* A surgical instrument used to cut and dissect tissue.

*Advanced Reference:* Scissors come in many shapes and sizes. They should be sharp in order to cleanly cut tissue and not tear it. The most commonly used scissors are Mcindoe, Mayo, Potts, Metzenbaum and iris, etc. Known as 'cut'.

**Sclerotherapy**   *Quick Reference:* (scler-row therapy) Injection of sclerosing agent to produce fibrosis.

*Advanced Reference:* Treatment used for *haemorrhoids, varicose veins* and oesophageal *varices.*

**Scoline**   *Quick Reference:* Depolarising skeletal-muscle relaxant.

*Advanced Reference:* Preparation of suxamethonium chloride. It has a duration of up to 5 min and commonly used for *intubation* in general anaesthesia (GA). *Fasiculation* occurs before paralysis is achieved. Also available as Anectine.

**Scoline apnoea** *Quick Reference:* Prolonged muscle paralysis.

*Advanced Reference:* Scoline *apnoea* occurs when the patient is given a depolarising muscle relaxant e.g. *suxamethonium*, if the patient is low on the enzyme cholinesterase which naturally breaks down the suxamethonium, the result is prolonged muscle paralysis (*scoline apnoea*). Treatment is to keep the patient sedated and ventilated until spontaneous reversal.

**Scopolamine** *Quick Reference:* Hyoscine.

*Advanced Reference:* A central nervous system (CNS) depressant. Has sedative, hypnotic and anti-emetic effects. Used as a premedication usually in combination with a narcotic. It is a more powerful drying agent (antisialogogue) than atropine.

**Screen** *Quick Reference:* Refers to the barrier device between the surgical and anaesthetic area of the operating table.

*Advanced Reference:* Also termed 'towel rail'. Has the intention of separating the sterile surgical field from the socially clean area of the anaesthetist as well as preventing drapes from covering the patient's face. A number of designs both home-made and manufactured are available. Jokingly referred to by anaesthetists as the 'blood–brain barrier'.

**Scrotum** *Quick Reference:* Pouch of skin below the root of the penis.

*Advanced Reference:* Contains the testes and accessory structures. Divided into two halves and the whole structure contracts in response to cold. Normally the testes themselves are placed so they are maintained at a slightly lower temperature than the rest of the body.

**Scrub area** *Quick Reference:* Area or room where theatre staff scrub prior to surgery.

*Advanced Reference:* Usually an anti-room to theatres or in some cases an area set aside for this purpose. Should be easily accessible but separate from general and patient entrances and exits.

**Secretions** *Quick Reference:* The formation by an organ/gland of a substance that is needed by some other organ or the body as a whole.

*Advanced Reference:* The secretions of exocrine glands are carried away in ducts or poured straight into the place where they are to be used, e.g. the secretion of the digestive glands and the glands of the skin. The secretions of endocrine glands (hormones) are released into the blood.

**Sedation** *Quick Reference:* The state of calming.

*Advanced Reference:* Involves the use of a sedative or tranquilliser, a drug which lessens excitement. Barbiturates and hypnotics are also used to produce sedation.

**See-saw breathing** *Quick Reference:* Also known as paradoxical breathing.

S

*Advanced Reference:* Seen in patients with airway obstruction. Upon observation, the chest falls as the abdomen rises when the patient attempts to breathe.

**Seldinger wire**   *Quick Reference:* (sell-ding-er) Device used to assist blood vessel catheterisation/cannulation.

*Advanced Reference:* A sprung wire originally used by radiologists and now adapted for venous/arterial cannulation/catheterisation. After venous access, the wire is fed through the cannula followed by the in-dwelling catheter being threaded over the wire. Upon successful catheterisation, the wire is removed. Wires now have at least one floppy end or in the shape of letter 'J' (*J-wire*) which eases passage through tortuous routes.

**Selectatec**   *Quick Reference:* (sell-ect-a-tech) Vaporiser-locking and securing system.

*Advanced Reference:* Only when the vaporiser is locked in position can gas enter. The system is also designed in a way that prevents two vaporisers being used simultaneously.

**Sellick's manoeuvre**   *Quick Reference:* (sell-licks) Manoeuvre carried out to prevent aspiration of stomach contents into the lungs.

*Advanced Reference:* Involves pressure being externally exerted on the *cricoid* cartilage during anaesthetic induction in an attempt to prevent regurgitated stomach contents entering the lungs. This is effective due to the cricoid cartilage being a circular structure and when depressed occludes the oesophagus. Utilised during emergency situations when a patient may not have been fasted, even with fasting still has the potential to have maintained gastric contents (*Caesarean section*), or when natural protection reflexes are insufficient (*hiatus hernia*). Named after the anaesthetist who first described its use. Also termed, crash induction, Rapid sequence induction.

**Semen**   *Quick Reference:* (see-men) The male genital (testicular) fluid.

*Advanced Reference:* Semen contains spermatozoa plus secretions of the prostate gland and seminal vesicles.

**Sengstaken-Blakemore tube**   *Quick Reference:* (Seng-starken) Multi-lumen device used for applying pressure to oesophageal varices.

*Advanced Reference:* The Minnesota tube is similar but has an extra lumen for oesophageal drainage. Both tubes have gastric and oesophageal balloons, which after oral insertion of the tube, are inflated and given traction in an effort to suppress bleeding.

**Septicaemia**   *Quick Reference:* The presence of bacterial toxins in the bloodstream. Blood poisoning.

*Advanced Reference:* Can lead to widespread tissue injury as the toxins are dispersed throughout the body by the bloodstream.

**Septum**   *Quick Reference:* A partition between two sides of a structure.

*Advanced Reference:* Example is the nasal septum, a sheet of cartilage between the nostrils and the interventricular septum dividing the two sides of the heart.

**Serum**   *Quick Reference:* The clear fluid that separates from whole blood when it clots.

*Advanced Reference:* It is plasma with fibrinogen removed and also contains antibodies and antitoxins.

**Servovent**   *Quick Reference:* (serve-o-vent) Name given to a type and design of patient ventilator.

*Advanced Reference:* The servomechanism is a control system applied to many ventilators but used to indicate certain ventilators, e.g. Manley Servovent and Siemens Servovent.

**Sesamoid**   *Quick Reference:* Bony mass said to resemble a sesame seed.

*Advanced Reference:* A small bony mass formed in tendons. The patella is the largest of the sesamoid bones.

**Set up room**   *Quick Reference:* A specific area for setting up of sterile instument trays.

*Advanced Reference:* Some theatre suites have an extra room adjacent to theatre which allows the scrub practitioner to prepare their sterile equipment. This is particularly helpful to promote the efficiency of a smooth running operating list.

**Sevoflurane**   *Quick Reference:* Volatile anaesthetic agent. Sometimes referred to as *servoflurane*.

*Advanced Reference:* One of the more recently introduced. Delivered via a vaporiser. Relatively insoluble so has a rapid induction and recovery action. Also suitable for gas induction in children due to its lack of irritating odour, as is the case with alternatives.

**Sharps**   *Quick Reference:* Refers to sharp items used in hospitals that have the potential to puncture, etc.

*Advanced Reference:* Items such as hypodermic needles, cannula needles, suture needles, scalpels or even large drain introducers and *laparoscopic* devices as well as glass. Under Control Of Substances Hazardous to Health (*COSHH*) Regulations, these must be disposed of in a designated container. These items pose many hazards with **needle-stick injury** being very common.

**Shelf-Life**   *Quick Reference:* Indicates the time within which an item should be used.

*Advanced Reference:* Corresponds to a 'sell by date'. In relation to operating departments, more usually involves sterile items and pharmaceuticals. Drugs may have their shelf-life extended with additives and preservatives and sterile adjuncts by the packaging method. As with industry etc, stock rotation should form a part of any theatre processes.

**Shock**  *Quick Reference:* Term used generally to indicate distress, etc. but in medical terms refers to a specific situation.

*Advanced Reference:* It is in fact a syndrome in which tissue perfusion is inadequate and leads to a number of signs and symptoms, e.g. *tachycardia, sweating, rapid-shallow breathing, hypotension.* Can be due to many causes and take many forms, i.e. anaphylactic shock, cardiogenic shock, septic shock, hypovolaemic shock, neurogenic shock, obstructive shock and distributive shock.

**Shunt**  *Quick Reference:* Diversion of flow, etc., as with circulation of blood.

*Advanced Reference:* In relation to haemodialysis, involves insertion of connecting tubing in adjacent artery and vein which can be used as access to the arterial and venous outlets of the artificial kidney machine.

**Sickle-cell anaemia**  *Quick Reference:* A genetically transmitted form of anaemia involving abnormal haemoglobin (Hb).

*Advanced Reference:* Under certain conditions including hypoxia, hypercarbia, hypothermia and acidosis, the abnormal Hb may distort (sickle) and rupture leading to blocking of small blood vessels and reduced oxygen-carrying capacity (haemolytic anaemia). Normal Hb is referred to as 'A', with abnormal termed 'S'. When the disease is inherited from both parents and almost all the Hb is abnormal, the condition is referred to as HbSS and when inherited from only one parent and there is a presence of both normal and abnormal Hb, this is termed HbAS. Known to mainly affect certain races such as those of Negroid background but now found in a broad range of the population.

**Sigmoidoscope**  *Quick Reference:* Device used to examine the lower bowel, etc.

*Advanced Reference:* Originally a rigid metal device with an externally fitted light source, long enough to view the sigmoid colon, rectum, etc. Now flexible versions are available with integrated light systems.

**Silastic**  *Quick Reference:* A rubbery silicone material.

*Advanced Reference:* Found in many medical products used in the operating room, e.g. breast implants.

**Silicone**  *Quick Reference:* Plastic-like material used in the manufacture of numerous medically related products.

*Advanced Reference:* An organic polymeric compound with many properties such as water resistant and passage of electricity. Also relatively inert to body actions and functions. Therefore, this lack of reaction enables devices to remain in the body for longer durations than plastics, i.e. feeding lines, oncology catheters, etc. Hence why many implants such as catheters, etc. are made from silicone.

**Silver nitrate**  *Quick Reference:* Substance used as a disinfectant and corrosive agent.

*Advanced Reference:* Seen primarily in the form of a stick used in the treatment of warts. Also used as an antiseptic in eye drops.

**Sino-atrial node**   *Quick Reference:* The natural pacemaker of the heart.
*Advanced Reference:* Situated in the atrium of the heart and instigates the heartbeat.

**Sinus**   *Quick Reference:* Indicates a pathway.
*Advanced Reference:* Indicates a hollow or cavity. There are a number of anatomical sinuses: brain, coronary, nasal, bone but also refers to a blind-ended opening or tract which usually starts from the body surface and becomes infected, etc.

**Sinus rhythm**   *Quick Reference:* Refers to the rhythm of the heart.
*Advanced Reference:* Sometimes referred to as normal rhythm (each P-wave is followed by a QRS-complex). Indicates the rhythm initiated by the *sino-atrial* node. *Sinus arrhythmia* is a condition where there are alternating phases of slow and rapid heart rates.

**Skin clips/staples**   *Quick Reference:* A sterile device used to close skin edges.
*Advanced Reference:* Made of non-corroding metal and originally applied with a non-disposable applicator. Gradually disposable automatic applicators were introduced. Skin clips/staples are quick and easy to insert and remove and leave a cosmetically acceptable scar.

**Sloops**   *Quick Reference:* Used during surgery to identify certain structures.
*Advanced Reference:* Come in various colours: red, blue, white and yellow. Sloops are used to identify structures, e.g. white for nerves, yellow for ureters, blue for veins and red for arteries; also the red and blue can be used to occlude vessels during vascular surgery.

**Smiths fracture**   *Quick Reference:* Fracture of the distal portion of the radius otherwise known as a reverse colles fracture.

**Sniffing the air**   *Quick Reference:* Refers to a head position in anaesthesia.
*Advanced Reference:* Actually termed 'sniffing the morning air'. Indicates when the head is flexed/extended for intubation.

**Soda lime**   *Quick Reference:* Mixture used for *carbon dioxide* ($CO_2$) absorption in anaesthetic-breathing systems.
*Advanced Reference:* Used to absorb the patients' exhaled $CO_2$. Composed of 94% calcium hydroxide, 5% sodium hydroxide and a trace of potassium hydroxide. Silica is added to prevent powdering of the granules and a dye is added to indicate when the soda lime is exhausted. Depending on variety in use, colour changes can be from white to violet or from pink to white.

**Sodium**   *Quick Reference:* Soft white element normally found in combination with other elements.

*Advanced Reference:* Essential for normal health and life, and forms the principal cation in the extracellular fluids. Commonly taken in the form of sodium chloride (common salt).

**Sodium bicarbonate**   *Quick Reference:* NaHCO$_3$ An ***alkali***.
*Advanced Reference:* Varying uses as an alkali and *antacid*. Most commonly seen during resuscitation when used in the treatment of *acidosis.*

**Sodium chloride**   *Quick Reference:* NaCl salt.
*Advanced Reference:* Widely used as saline solution (normal saline is 0.9%) as a replacement and maintenance intravenous (IV) fluid. Also used as an irrigating solution in urology following endoscopic bladder procedures.

**Sodium citrate**   *Quick Reference:* Alkaline compound used to treat infections of the urinary tract.
*Advanced Reference:* Also used to assist in the secretion of uric acid.

**Sodium hypochlorite**   *Quick Reference:* Used as a disinfectant.
*Advanced Reference:* Mainly used for cleaning abrasions, etc. Available in 1% and 8% concentrations.

**Sodium lactate**   *Quick Reference:* Hartmanns solution.
*Advanced Reference:* Crystalloid solution. IV replacement and maintenance fluid.

**Soft palate**   *Quick Reference:* Posterior portion of the roof of the mouth.
*Advanced Reference:* The soft palate extends from the palatine bones to the *uvula*.

**Solu-Cortef**   *Quick Reference:* Proprietary corticosteroid (***hydrocortisone***).
*Advanced Reference:* Used to replace steroid deficiency, suppress inflammation or allergic symptoms or to treat shock. Produced in powder form for reconstitution.

**Solu-Medrone**   *Quick Reference:* Proprietary corticosteroid, e.g. methyl-prednisolone.
*Advanced Reference:* Used to treat shock and suppress allergic and inflammatory symptoms.

**Solution**   *Quick Reference:* Liquid in which a substance is dissolved.
*Advanced Reference:* A fluid which contains a dissolved substance (solute).

**Sotalol**   *Quick Reference:* ***Beta-blocker*** and antihypertensive.
*Advanced Reference:* Used to treat hypertension, arrhythmias and angina.

**Spatula**   *Quick Reference:* A flat blunt-edged instrument.
*Advanced Reference:* Seen commonly as a *tongue-depressor* made of metal or wood.

**Specimens**  *Quick Reference:* Indicates a sample taken from a body part or area.

*Advanced Reference:* Specimens are taken to determine their nature and/or the presence of disease, etc. Depending on the tissue involved and the examination required, specimens are placed in various containers and mediums. Examples include blood, cells, tissue, fluid, pus, etc.

**Speculum**  *Quick Reference:* An instrument for inspecting the interior of natural body passages.

*Advanced Reference:* Often fitted with illumination or mirrors. Has a limited usage in terms of an *endoscope*, so used for viewing relatively peripheral areas. Speculums are available for viewing, the vagina, rectum, nose, outer ear.

**Spermicidal**  *Quick Reference:* Substances which kill sperm.

*Advanced Reference:* Not a contraceptive in themselves but are used in barrier methods such as condoms and creams.

**Sphincter**  *Quick Reference:* A ring of muscle.

*Advanced Reference:* Has the ability to constrict and close a natural passage or close an orifice, e.g. anal sphincter, gastro-oesophageal sphincter.

**Sphygmomanometer**  *Quick Reference:* (spig-mom-an-om-eater)) Instrument for measuring the blood pressure (BP) (non-invasive).

*Advanced Reference:* Indicates an external gauge which records the pressure of air needed to stop the flow of blood into a limb.

**Spinal**  *Quick Reference:* Term used to describe spinal anaesthesia. Intradural.

*Advanced Reference:* Involves the passage of a fine needle into the subarachnoid space (cerebrospinal fluid, *CSF*) followed by injection of local anaesthetic (LA) to bring about loss of pain.

**Spirometer**  *Quick Reference:* Device used to measure lung volumes.

*Advanced Reference:* Various types exist, those which involve moving a cylinder up a column or dial with a needle, etc. Used during anaesthesia and generally for investigative reasons. Examples are the vitalograph and *Wright's respirometer*.

**Sponge holder**  *Quick Reference:* Surgical instrument for holding small swabs.

*Advanced Reference:* Involves wrapping a small (4 × 4) swab around the end of the instrument (Rampleys) and used for prepping, retraction and swabbing, etc. Also referred to as *'swab on a stick'*.

**Static**  *Quick Reference:* With reference to theatres indicates static electricity.

*Advanced Reference:* Involves the build-up of an electrical charge in a non-conductor. In theatres, this can be caused by two unlike surfaces rubbing together as with patient clothing and operating table covers, etc.

Can lead to sparking which has the possibility of igniting with support from gases and vapours. It was standard at one time for *carbon* to be included as a conductor in many pieces of theatre equipment.

**Stemetil**    *Quick Reference:* Proprietary anti-emetic, e.g. prochlorperazine.

*Advanced Reference:* Used to treat nausea. Used as a post-operative anti-emetic and for the nausea caused by vertigo, inner ear infections, etc.

**Stent**    *Quick Reference:* Device used as a support or splint.

*Advanced Reference:* Stents are used in urology to maintain patency of the ureters. Also utilised in ophthalmology, vascular surgery, in the oesophagus or bile duct, etc. Placed across an obstruction to maintain an open lumen or as support after creation of an *anastomosis*.

**Stereotaxy**    *Quick Reference:* (sterio-taxi) An intracranial approach using accurate geometric calculations to set a target in order to obtain biopsies or perform a specialised neurosurgical procedure.

*Advanced Reference:* Predetermined anatomical landmarks are used as guides. Special head fixation devices have been developed for use with radiography, fluoroscopy, computerised tomography (CT) scans and magnetic resonance imaging (MRI) to permit accurate placement of a probe directed at the target area.

**Sterile field**    *Quick Reference:* Indicates an area that has been made free from contamination.

*Advanced Reference:* In theatres refers to the area including the patient and scrub staff that has been made aseptic by the use of washing, drap-ing, screening, etc. Also directly refers to the area of a patient or sur-rounding area prepared for a sterile procedure.

**Sterilisation**    *Quick Reference:* Actually indicates the inability to reproduce.

*Advanced Reference:* Although can be used to indicate certain proced-ures, such as vasectomy, tubal ligation or clipping, it is generally used to indicate the process of ridding articles free of bacteria, etc. This is done with the use of autoclaves/ovens (heat), chemicals, gases and irradiation.

**Sternal notch**    *Quick Reference:* Anatomical landmark found at the top of the sternum.

*Advanced Reference:* Notch in the top of the sternum found below the cricoid area.

**Sternomastoid**    *Quick Reference:* Large muscle at the side of the neck.

*Advanced Reference:* The muscle extends from the top of the sternum and clavicle to the skull behind the ear. It facilitates flexing of the head and rotation of the neck. Also a common landmark during CVP cannulation.

**Sternum**    *Quick Reference:* Breast bone.

*Advanced Reference:* Flat bone at the front of the chest to which the upper ribs are attached. The upper part, or manubrium, slopes downwards and forwards making an angle with the vertical body section. A joint between manubrium and body allows the sternum to straighten when the ribs rise during inspiration.

**Steroids**   *Quick Reference:* Naturally occurring and synthetic agents based on sterone.

*Advanced Reference:* In the body they include *hormones* of the adrenal cortex and sex glands (e.g. *oestrogens*).

**Stethoscope**   *Quick Reference:* Instrument used to listen to interior body sounds.

*Advanced Reference:* Used mainly for listening to heart and lungs. Invented by a French physician. Traditionally consists of listening attachments fitted to rubber tubing, but variation are available for listening to foetal heartbeat in the uterus (manual and electronic) as well as *oesophageal stethoscopes* used during anaesthesia.

**Stoma**   *Quick Reference:* A mouth-like opening.

*Advanced Reference:* Usually refers to an artificial opening made in the skin surface as a collection point for various internal anatomy, e.g. colostomy and ileostomy.

**Stomach**   *Quick Reference:* That part of the digestive tract between the lower end of the oesophagus and the beginning of the intestine.

*Advanced Reference:* The first part of the stomach is the *fundus*, which forms a dome under the left side of the diaphragm. The second part, the body, broadens out and runs down from the fundus to the third part, the antrum, which is funnel shaped and runs upwards to the right and ends in the midline of the body at the pylorus, a muscular tube acting as a valve between the stomach and the duodenum.

**Streptokinase**   *Quick Reference:* (strep-toe-ki-an-ase) *Enzyme* used therapeutically as a fibrinolytic drug, e.g. streptase.

*Advanced Reference:* Used to break down blood clots, useful in the treatment of *thrombosis* and *embolism*.

**Streptomycin**   *Quick Reference: Antibiotic.*

*Advanced Reference:* Mostly used now in the treatment of tuberculosis (TB) and usually in combination with other antibiotics.

**Stridor**   *Quick Reference:* Noise of the respiratory tract.

*Advanced Reference:* Noise made by the breath passing an obstruction in the larynx or trachea.

**Stripper**   *Quick Reference:* A surgical instrument used for removal of varicose veins.

*Advanced Reference:* Made of flexible sometimes sprung metal with a removable cone-shaped end (choc). The wire is threaded down the vein (long saphenous), then the choc attached and pulled back up the vein and so stripping out the vein from surrounding tissue.

**Stroke**   *Quick Reference:* Sudden interference with the circulation of blood to a part of the brain. A CVA (Cerebrovascular accident).
*Advanced Reference:* Also termed *apoplexy*. Caused by a sudden accident (haemorrhage, thrombosis or embolism) occurring in a blood vessel responsible for part of the blood supply to the brain, resulting in unconsciousness, paralysis or death.

**Stylette**   *Quick Reference:* (Sti-let) Endotracheal (ET) tube introducer.
*Advanced Reference:* A *malleable* introducer designed to assist re-shaping of the ET tube in the event of difficult intubation. Made from various materials including copper, plastic-coated metal, etc.

**Subarachnoid**   *Quick Reference:* Fluid-filled space between the coverings of the brain and spinal cord.
*Advanced Reference:* The subarachnoid space lies beneath the arachnoid membrane and pia mater of the brain and contains *CSF.*

**Subclavian**   *Quick Reference:* Under the *collarbone* (clavicle).
*Advanced Reference:* Both the subclavian artery and vein accompany each other below the clavicle. The vein regularly used for central venous pressure (**CVP**) insertion.

**Sublimaze**   *Quick Reference:* Fentanyl. **Narcotic** analgesic.
*Advanced Reference:* Synthetic analgesic derived from *pethidine* and commonly used for intra-operative analgesia. In small doses lasts approximately 30 min but in large doses can have a duration of 2–3 hours. Powerful respiratory depressant but has virtually no cardiovascular effects.

**Suction**   *Quick Reference:* Indicates a suction device.
*Advanced Reference:* General term to indicate a suction machine for use in surgery and anaesthesia rather than the actual act of suctioning.

**Sufentanil**   *Quick Reference:* Synthetic opioid analgesic drug.
*Advanced Reference:* A relative of fentanyl with similar effects but less potent and has a shorter elimination period.

**Sulphonamides**   *Quick Reference:* (sul-fon-a-mides) Literally a sulpha drug.
*Advanced Reference:* Drugs that prevent the growth of bacteria. Often confused with antibiotics but are in fact a distinct group and in some cases may be used as an alternative where there may be adverse side effects.

**Sump drain**   *Quick Reference:* A double-lumen surgical wound drain.
*Advanced Reference:* Made of plastic or rubber and used to remove accumulated fluids from cavities. Can be used with or without suction.

**Supine**   *Quick Reference:* (Soo-pine) Patients positioned on their back.
*Advanced Reference:* When patients are in a supine position they are flat on their back. This is the most common position for patients in the operating department.

**Suprapubic**   *Quick Reference:* Indicates above the pubic bone.
*Advanced Reference:* Used in relation to a number of procedures. Suprapubic cystotomy is making an incision into the urinary bladder. Suprapubic *prostatectomy* indicates the removal of the gland by an approach from above the pubic bone, as opposed to the *trans-urethral* approach.

**Surfactant**   *Quick Reference:* Lubricating agent.
*Advanced Reference: Pulmonary* surfactant is secreted by the alveoli lowering surface tension and so allowing free expansion of the chest wall. Absence of surfactant can lead to *respiratory distress syndrome.*

**Surgicel**   *Quick Reference:* Surgical haemostatic agent.
*Advanced Reference:* Oxidised cellulose, reacts with the body tissues and swells to form a seal over the area that is bleeding.

**Suture**   *Quick Reference:* A stitch used to close a wound or a junction between two bones as in the *cranium* and **occipital** regions.
*Advanced Reference:* More commonly indicates the device used to close or repair during surgery. Made in numerous sizes and from varying materials to suit need, use and specific tissue. May be natural or synthetic, absorbable or non-absorbable, mono-filament or multi-filament. Suturing describes the act of sewing, methods and styles vary and can be *continuous* or *non-continuous.* Attached needles are also designed to suit need, being blunt, cutting, round bodied and of varying shapes, curved, straight, etc.

**Swabs**   *Quick Reference:* An item used to absorb blood.
*Advanced Reference:* Besides being used to absorb blood at a wound or operation site, swabs are used to pack cavities and aid blunt dissection. Usually made of cotton, gauze, they are available in a range of sizes and designs. Surgical swabs come in large sizes (abdo-packs) down to small (4 × 4s) as well as *pledgets* and *patties* for more finer and speciality purposes. All swabs that are to enter the body cavity have some form of detection system if mislaid, e.g. ray-tec strip. Swab-count indicates the process used to record the number of swabs prepared and used during surgery.

**Swan–Ganz catheter**   *Quick Reference:* Balloon-tipped, *multi-lumen catheter* used to measure pulmonary artery pressures.
*Advanced Reference:* Also termed pulmonary artery and flotation catheter. Via venous access, the catheter is floated into the right atrium onto the right ventricle and eventually pulmonary artery in order to obtain pressure readings for diagnosis of ventricular function and output performance.

**Symphysis pubis**   *Quick Reference:* The cartilaginous junction of the two pubic bones.

*Advanced Reference:* A symphysis is a cartilaginous joint along the line of the union of two bones.

**Synovial**   *Quick Reference:* Indicates the area incorporating a joint.

*Advanced Reference:* Synovial fluid is the lubricating fluid secreted by the synovial membrane to act as a lubricant for the joint. Synovitis is inflammation of the membrane.

**Syntocinon**   *Quick Reference:* (sin-toe-sin-on) Proprietary preparation of the hormone oxytocin.

*Advanced Reference:* Causes increased contraction of the uterus during labour. Administered therapeutically to induce or assist labour and control postnatal bleeding. Used in similar circumstances to *ergometrine.*

**Syntometrine**   *Quick Reference:* (sin-toe-met-rine) A proprietary preparation of the alkaloid ergometrine together with oxytocin. Similar effects and use to *ergometrine* and *syntocinon.*

*Advanced Reference:* Used during the final stages of labour and control postnatal bleeding.

**Syringe pump**   *Quick Reference:* Programmed pumps that can be adjusted to deliver differing rates of infusion.

*Advanced Reference:* Utilised in *anaesthesia,* intensive care units (ICUs) and throughout mainly *critical-care* areas. Numerous designs exist and in some cases for specific use. Involve the mounting of a syringe to a motorised driver system. Commonly used for patient-controlled analgesia (PCA), drug infusion, etc.

**Systole**   *Quick Reference:* Contraction period of the heart muscle.

*Advanced Reference:* Atrial systole (contraction) is the phase when blood is pumped from the atria to the ventricles and ventricular systole (contraction) involves the pumping of blood into the aorta and pulmonary artery.

# T

**Tachycardia** *Quick Reference:* (tac-e-card-ea) Rapid heartbeat. Tachy indicates fast or rapid.

*Advanced Reference:* May be due to many causes: fever, emotion, exercise, infection, pain, anaemia, haemorrhage, drugs or disorder of the cardiac rhythm.

**Tamponade** *Quick Reference:* (tam-pon-ard) Abnormal pressure on part of the body affecting function.

*Advanced Reference:* Example would be cardiac tamponade when the presence of fluid, e.g. blood, between the *pericardium* and the heart causes excessive pressure.

**Tare weight** *Quick Reference:* Empty weight.

*Advanced Reference:* Marking on a nitrous oxide cylinder to indicate the weight of the empty cylinder due to the contents being liquid and not a gas. Can be weighed to ascertain contents.

**Tarsus** *Quick Reference:* Base of the foot. Of the seven tarsal bones only one, the talus articulates with the leg to form the ankle joint.

*Advanced Reference:* Alternatively, it is the flat firm plate of connective tissue which supports the eyelid.

**Temazepam** *Quick Reference:* Short-acting *benzodiazepine*.

*Advanced Reference:* Often used in cases of insomnia and regularly as a premedication before general anaesthesia (GA).

**Temgesic** *Quick Reference:* Narcotic analgesic.

*Advanced Reference:* Used to treat all forms of pain. It is a preparation of the *opiate* buprenorphine hydrochloride.

**Temporo-mandibular joint** *Quick Reference:* Joint between the temporal bone of the skull and the lower jaw.

*Advanced Reference:* The joint lies just in front of the ear and is of sliding hinge design which allows movement of the mandible from side to side and the two bones are separated by a plate of cartilage inside the joint. Stiffness, deformity or injury to this joint may lead to difficult intubation.

T

**Tendon**   *Quick Reference:* Sinew.
*Advanced Reference:* Cord structure made of dense fibrous tissue which joins muscle to bone.

**Tenotomy**   *Quick Reference:* Surgical division of a tendon.
*Advanced Reference:* An operative procedure of the tendon to correct a deformity caused by its shortening. Also an ophthalmology procedure to correct a squint.

**Termination**   *Quick Reference:* Commonly used to indicate termination of pregnancy.
*Advanced Reference:* Indicates abortion, usually surgical but can include methods using drugs, etc.

**Test dose**   *Quick Reference:* Administration of a small amount of a drug.
*Advanced Reference:* Term applied to injection of local anaesthetic (LA) in epidural procedures. A small dose of drug is given before the main dose in order to identify accidental *subarachnoid* or intravenous (IV) injection via the epidural catheter. A similar system is also carried out with certain antibiotics to determine allergic response.

**Testosterone**   *Quick Reference:* Male sex hormone being the principal hormone of the testis.
*Advanced Reference:* It is necessary for the development of the secondary sexual characteristics, i.e. beard growth, pubic hair, enlargement of genital organs, lowering of the voice at puberty together with change in body shape at puberty. Also responsible for the production of semen.

**Tetanus**   *Quick Reference:* Acute disease of the nervous system.
*Advanced Reference:* Caused by the micro-organism *Clostridium tetani*, mainly due to contamination from soil. Initially, muscle stiffness occurs around the site of the wound then followed by rigidity of the face and neck muscles and the mouth will not open fully (*lock jaw*). Prevention is by active immunisation with tetanus toxoid. Booster doses are given at recommended intervals.

**Tetracyclines**   *Quick Reference:* (tet-ra-sice-lean) Antibiotic group of drugs.
*Advanced Reference:* They have broad-spectrum activity but many organisms have developed resistance to them but they are still used to treat *Chlamydia* and *Rickettsia*. Tetracyclines are deposited in growing bones and teeth, staining them yellow and are therefore not given to pregnant women, those breastfeeding or children under 12.

**Thalamonal**   *Quick Reference:* A proprietary preparation of fentanyl and *droperidol*.
*Advanced Reference:* This combination of a tranquilliser and narcotic analgesic may be used for patients undergoing diagnostic or minor surgical procedures.

**Thalamus**  *Quick Reference:* Two masses of nerve cells positioned at the base of the *cerebrum*.

*Advanced Reference:* Sensations of all kinds are carried to the thalamus and then relayed to the cerebral cortex where they are perceived. If the thalamus is damaged, the perception of pain sensation can be affected.

**Thalassaemia**  *Quick Reference:* (thal-a-seem-ea) An inherited defect in the formation of *haemoglobin* (Hb).

*Advanced Reference:* There are a number of types classified as major through to minor. The severest sometimes leading to death occurring before adolescence and the minor forms displaying few symptoms. Mostly found in Mediterranean regions and passed on from parents to children.

**Theophylline**  *Quick Reference:* (thee-off-eline) A drug which dilates the bronchi.

*Advanced Reference:* Derived from tea leaves or made synthetically is used in the treatment of *asthma* and *bronchospasm*.

**Therapeutics**  *Quick Reference:* (ther-a-putic) The study of the science of treating disease.

*Advanced Reference:* Therapy is the treatment of disease.

**Therm**  *Quick Reference:* Unit of heat.

*Advanced Reference:* Thermal indicates a relationship to heat.

**Thermistor**  *Quick Reference:* Device involved in temperature measurement.

*Advanced Reference:* Found in clinical temperature probes and pulmonary artery (PA) catheters for measuring cardiac output. Involves a semiconductor whose resistance changes with temperature.

**Thermocouple**  *Quick Reference:* Device involved in temperature measurement.

*Advanced Reference:* Involves two strips of dissimilar metals which expand at different temperatures. The metals expand and contract in response to temperature changes and produce an electrical potential that then makes reference to pre-settings. Found in *autoclaves*.

**Thiazides**  *Quick Reference:* (thia-zides) Diuretic group of drugs.

*Advanced Reference:* Thiazides act on the first part of the convoluted tubule in the kidney blocking the re-absorption of *sodium*. Used in the treatment of high blood pressure (BP) and heart failure.

**Thiopentone**  *Quick Reference:* IV anaesthetic agent.

*Advanced Reference:* Short-acting barbiturate used in a 2.5% solution in the UK. Alternatively named *sodium pentothal* or *intraval sodium*. Referred to as the 'truth drug' in the US. Also used as an anticonvulsive. Stored as a yellow powder and reconstituted with water when required. Gives off a garlic smell and taste due to the sulphur content. Effects may endure for up to 24 hours after administration.

**Thomas splint**  *Quick Reference:* Splint used to immobilise knee, femur, etc.
*Advanced Reference:* The shape and design of this splint supports the limb as well as moving the weight from the knee joint to the *pelvis*. Named after the British orthopaedic surgeon, Hugh Thomas.

**Thoracic duct**  *Quick Reference:* The large lymph vessel that begins at the cisterna chyli which is a sac lying adjacent to the aorta in the aortic opening of the diaphragm. Into this drains the right and left lumbar lymph trunks draining the lower limbs and intestinal trunk. From here the thoracic duct runs up through the thorax to the neck and comes to lie on the right side of the oesophagus. The lymph carried by the thoracic duct runs into the *subclavian* vein.

**Thoracoscopy**  *Quick Reference:* Inspection of the interior of the chest through an *endoscope*.
*Advanced Reference:* More specifically involves examination of the pleural cavity as well as the thoracic cavity.

**Thoracotomy**  *Quick Reference:* The surgical opening of the wall of the chest.
*Advanced Reference:* Any surgical operation that involves opening the thorax.

**Thorax**  *Quick Reference:* The chest compartment.
*Advanced Reference:* The thorax is enclosed by the ribs, reaching from the first rib to the diaphragm.

**Throat spray**  *Quick Reference:* Refers to an LA throat spray used in anaesthesia.
*Advanced Reference:* Used after induction and/or muscle relaxation to decrease the stimulus and presence of the endotracheal (ET) tube by coating the laryngeal and tracheal mucosa with (usually 4%) lignocaine. Originally delivered via a refillable Macintosh and Forrester spray but more recently a preloaded sealed unit has been available.

**Throb**  *Quick Reference:* To beat or pulsate.
*Advanced Reference:* Felt in the presence of infection when the area is said to throb.

**Thrombin**  *Quick Reference:* An enzyme involved in the coagulation of blood.
*Advanced Reference:* Thrombin converts fibrinogen to fibrin during the blood-clotting process.

**Thrombophlebitis**  *Quick Reference:* (throm-bo-fle-bitis) Inflammation of a vein with consequent thrombosis.
*Advanced Reference:* With reference to theatre patients, it is commonly associated with post-operative IV cannula sites. Involves clotting at the site combined with inflammation of the lining of the vessel.

**Thrombosis**    *Quick Reference:* Formation of a clot or thrombus in a blood vessel.

*Advanced Reference:* May occur in arteries when the walls have been roughened by *atherosclerosis* or in veins when the circulation becomes sluggish or stagnant.

**Thrombus**    *Quick Reference:* Thrombosis is formation of a blood clot within a vessel.

*Advanced Reference:* Indicates a blood clot that formed within the vessel (usually a vein) and is stationary. Once it moves from its original site, it is termed an *embolus*.

**Thymol**    *Quick Reference:* A mild antiseptic derived from oil of thyme.

*Advanced Reference:* A hydrocarbon also used as an anti-oxidant in some volatile agents. Other uses are as a disinfectant, mouthwash and deodorant.

**Thymus**    *Quick Reference:* (thi-mus) Gland which lies at the root of the neck behind the breastbone in the upper mediastinum.

*Advanced Reference:* The gland grows from birth to puberty and thereafter diminishes in size but remains active. It is an important part of the lymphatic system being responsible for the formation of lymphocytes (T-cells) which are essential in the immune reaction.

**Thyroid**    *Quick Reference:* A ductless gland lying in the neck.

*Advanced Reference:* The thyroid lies at the front of the neck in front of the *trachea* and just below the *larynx*. It has two lobes and secretes two hormones, thyroxine being the most prominent. Swelling of the gland is known as goitre and normal function of the gland depends on an adequate intake of *iodine* in the diet.

**Thyrotoxicosis**    *Quick Reference:* (thyro-tox-i-cosis) Overactivity of the thyroid gland.

*Advanced Reference:* Also termed hyperthyroidism. Involves enlargement of the gland and a speeding up of metabolism resulting in nervousness, sweating, emotional overactivity, loss of weight, etc.

**TIA**    *Quick Reference:* Transient ischaemic attack. Minor stroke.

*Advanced Reference:* Involves numbness in the affected part, face, arm, etc.; sometimes with speech disturbance, *nausea*, double vision but not usually loss of consciousness. It is due to small clots partially blocking arteries in the brain and connected nerves lose function temporarily unlike with a major stroke where there is no return of function. However, TIAs may indicate future *stroke*.

**Tibia**    *Quick Reference:* The shin bone.

*Advanced Reference:* One of the two parallel bones in the lower leg and extends from the knee to the ankle. Corresponding with the radius in the forearm. The tibia is much more heavily built as it carries all the body weight.

**Tidal volume**  *Quick Reference:* Volume of air that moves into the lungs with each inspiration.

*Advanced Reference:* Tidal volume (TV) is used in relation to minute volume (MV) and respiratory rate (RR). MV = TV × RR.

**Tincture**  *Quick Reference:* An alcoholic solution of a drug/medicine, etc.

*Advanced Reference:* Commonly seen in theatres as tincture of iodine, alcoholic *chlorhexidine* (hibitane), etc., more so than drug preparations.

**Tinnitus**  *Quick Reference:* (tin-nit-tus) Noises in the ears.

*Advanced Reference:* May be buzzing, ringing, hissing, whistling and may follow disease of the *auditory* nerve or *cochlea*.

**Tissue fluid**  *Quick Reference:* Also termed extracellular fluid.

*Advanced Reference:* Watery fluid percolating all the minute spaces of/ between the body cells.

**Tissue forceps**  *Quick Reference:* An instrument used for grasping tissue during surgery.

*Advanced Reference:* There are numerous types and design, among the most commonly used are Allis, Lanes, Babcock and Duvals.

**Titanium**  *Quick Reference:* Grey metallic element.

*Advanced Reference:* Used in many implants such as hips. Has many desirable properties, i.e. low solubility, strong, non-toxic, non-carcinogenic and non-irritant.

**TIVA**  *Quick Reference:* Total IV anaesthesia. Technique which uses only IV drugs.

*Advanced Reference:* Aimed at avoiding the use of inhalation agents and usually given via infusion. Has the benefits of avoiding pollution and the unwanted effects of inhalation agents.

**Tobramycin**  *Quick Reference:* Antibiotic. Tobralex.

*Advanced Reference:* Effective against many forms of bacteria as well as a range of other micro-organisms.

**Tomography**  *Quick Reference:* (tomogram) X-ray intended to show structures lying in a selected plane on the body.

*Advanced Reference:* Can involve the use of X-rays or ultrasound waves in order to view a layer of body tissue irrespective of depth.

**Tonic**  *Quick Reference:* Refers to tension or pressure.

*Advanced Reference:* Tonicity can be applied to fluids in terms of their *osmotic* pressure, also muscles when they are in a state of continuous contraction as opposed to the normal situation of contraction and relaxation.

**Tonsils**  *Quick Reference:* A mass of lymphoid tissue.

*Advanced Reference:* Two lymph glands situated in the back of the throat between the pillars of fauces which forms part of **Waldeyer's Ring**.

**Topical anaesthesia**  *Quick Reference:* Surface application of LA.

*Advanced Reference:* Applied to skin, mucous membrane (pharynx, nasal passages, urethra, conjunctiva), etc. via direct application, swabs, pastes, sprays.

**Torecan**  *Quick Reference:* Proprietary anti-emetic.

*Advanced Reference:* Used to relieve nausea and vomiting. Torecan is a preparation of thiethylperazine.

**Toronto frame**  *Quick Reference:* Piece of patient positioning equipment.

*Advanced Reference:* Also referred to as the Montreal frame among other descriptions. Used as support with the patient laying face-down on the frame during spinal surgery.

**Tourniquet**  *Quick Reference:* (turn-i-kay) A constrictive band placed tightly around a limb to stop the flow of blood.

*Advanced Reference:* The intention is to compress both arteries and veins while the purpose can be varied, i.e. to stop arterial bleeding from a wound, prevent the spread of venom or poison, or provide a surgeon with a bloodless field. In relation to theatres, numerous designs exist and guidelines with regard to pressures and times vary according to local policy. The position, pressure being used and time duration applied are of utmost importance irrespective of purpose.

**Toxaemia**  *Quick Reference:* Blood poisoning.

*Advanced Reference:* This occurs due to an underlying bacterial infection within the body.

**Toxin**  *Quick Reference:* A poison. Toxic means poisonous.

*Advanced Reference:* Toxicology is the study of poisons and their actions. The source of the toxin may be varied but used commonly to indicate those of bacterial or animal origin. Toxoid refers to modified bacterial toxins that have lost their poisonous properties but can still act as antigens to provoke the formation of *antibodies* but does not produce symptoms of the disease. **Tetanus** toxoid is used to induce immunity to tetanus.

**TPN**  *Quick Reference:* Total parenteral nutrition.

*Advanced Reference:* Involves the giving of nutrition via a vein in cases where the patient is unable to take or absorb food by the **enteral** route because of obstruction, bowel removal, unconsciousness/coma, etc.

**Trachea**  *Quick Reference:* The windpipe.

*Advanced Reference:* The trachea runs from the larynx downwards into the upper mediastinum and divides into the right and left main bronchi.

**Tracheostomy**   *Quick Reference:* (track-e-ostomy) A surgical procedure for establishing an airway.

*Advanced Reference:* Involves entering the trachea through a hole made in the neck at approximately the level of the third tracheal ring. Carried out for numerous reasons, i.e. obstruction, long-term ventilation, laryngectomy, etc. followed by insertion of a tracheostomy tube which can be permanent or temporary depending on the cause.

**Tracrium**   *Quick Reference:* Non-depolarising muscle relaxant.

*Advanced Reference:* Atracurium, muscle relaxant with short duration, useful with renal and liver failure patients as it does not require their function for elimination.

**Train of four (ToF)**   *Quick Reference:* Refers to nerve stimulation with muscular blockade.

*Advanced Reference:* In relation to peripheral nerve stimulators, ToF is used to monitor the degree of neuromuscular block. The ToF ratio compares the fourth to first twitch produced by the stimulator.

**Tramadol**   *Quick Reference:* Opioid analgesic, e.g. zydol.

*Advanced Reference:* Reported to have fewer of the typical opioid side effects, notably, less respiratory depression, reduced constipation action and less addiction potential.

**Tranquillisers**   *Quick Reference:* Group of drugs used to sedate and allay anxiety.

*Advanced Reference:* Designed to have a general calming effect in numerous situations and conditions. They have been divided into a number of classes, the major being used to treat psychotic states and the minor in severe cases of anxiety and as aids to sleep. Minor tranquillisers are also known as anxiolytics and major drugs called antipsychotics or neuroleptics.

**Transducer**   *Quick Reference:* Device that changes one energy form into another.

*Advanced Reference:* Commonly used in theatre for invasive pressure monitoring. Transducers convert one form of energy into another, i.e. mechanical energy into an electrical impulse.

**Transfusion**   *Quick Reference:* The transfer of blood.

*Advanced Reference:* From one human to another through a vein. Used to replace actual volume or various blood products. *Auto-transfusion* is the use of a persons' own blood. Exchange or replacement transfusion is the removal or replacement of all or most of a recipient's blood. Direct transfusion involves the direct transfer from ***donor*** to ***recipient***.

**Translucent**   *Quick Reference:* Shining, clear.
*Advanced Reference:* Any medium through which light can pass but in a diffused manner.

**Transplantation**   *Quick Reference:* Transfer of tissue or organ from one subject to another unlike grafting which is used to indicate moving tissue from one part to another of the same person.
*Advanced Reference:* Transplantation is now regularly used for hearts, lungs, kidneys, pancreas, bone, cornea, etc. Donor being the source of the organ or part to be transplanted and recipient indicating the one receiving the donor part.

**Transposition**   *Quick Reference:* A developmental fault in relation to the heart.
*Advanced Reference:* Involves the **aorta** arising from the right side of the heart instead of the left and the *PA* (pulmonary artery) from the left instead of the right. **Dextrocardia** involves a mirror image to normal with the apex of the heart being towards the right.

**Trans-urethral resection of prostate**   *Quick Reference:* TURP, reduction or removal of the prostate gland via an endoscope.
*Advanced Reference:* Also termed *trans-urethral retrograde prostatectomy.* Involves the excision of the prostate using a resectoscope passed via the urethra into the bladder.
An alternative operation is open prostatectomy (*retropubic* and *transvesical*) the approach being via a lower abdominal incision. TURT is trans-urethral resection of tumour and TURBN is trans-urethral resection of bladder neck.

**Trauma**   *Quick Reference:* An injury or wound.
*Advanced Reference:* Can be applied to both physical and mental situations. Physical indicates injury and or damage to body tissues, etc.

**Trendelenburg**   *Quick Reference:* Operation and position. Now most commonly used with reference to an operating table position.
*Advanced Reference:* Trendelenburg position is head down with the body sloping downwards and backwards. Used now for a number of procedures but originally for the operation of varicose veins and named after the German surgeon, Freidrich Trendelenburg. In the original position the knees were bent and hanging down at about 40°.

**Trephine**   *Quick Reference:* (tref-ine) Surgical instrument.
*Advanced Reference:* Used mainly in neurosurgical operations as an instrument for removing a circle or disc of bone in the skull. A trepan is a cylindrical saw used for the same purpose. A similar instrument is used in *ophthalmics* to cut out a piece of **cornea**.

**Triage**   *Quick Reference:* To sort, sift or filter.

*Advanced Reference:* Classifying patients according to severity of injuries. Used in major accident scenes, accident and emergency (A&E) departments, etc.

**Tricuspid**   *Quick Reference:* Having three cusps or flaps.
*Advanced Reference:* The tricuspid valve is situated between the right atrium and right ventricle of the heart.

**Tricyclic antidepressants**   *Quick Reference:* (try-sice-lic) Class of antidepressant drugs.
*Advanced Reference:* These are used in more serious cases of depression. Side effects include *arrhythmias*, *heart block* and *convulsions*.

**Tridil**   *Quick Reference:* Vasodilator drug.
*Advanced Reference:* Used to treat *angina pectoris*. Available in ampoules for injection/infusion as glyceryl trinitrate (GTN).

**Trigeminal nerve**   *Quick Reference:* Fifth cranial nerve.
*Advanced Reference:* Sensory nerve of the face. It has three divisions: *ophthalmic*, *maxillary*, *mandibular* or first, second, third, as well as a motor branch which supplies the muscles used in chewing.

**Trigeminy**   *Quick Reference:* (try-gem-ine) Irregular pulse or heartbeat.
*Advanced Reference:* Involves an ECG trace when there are three beats then a missed beat. Refers to heartbeats in groups of three, e.g. premature ectopics.

**Trilene**   *Quick Reference:* (try-lean) Trichloroethylene. Volatile anaesthetic agent.
*Advanced Reference:* No longer available. Inhalation agent with analgesic properties once used regularly in anaesthetic practice, especially obstetrics, where it was also used during labour in a device called a Tritec. Not to be used with soda lime in a closed circuit as it produces toxic metabolites which cause cranial nerve damage. Used in industry as a dry-cleaning fluid and solvent.

**Trimetaphan**   *Quick Reference:* (tri-met-a-fan) Drug that reduces BP.
*Advanced Reference:* Technically a hypotensive agent with short duration. Used in many types of surgery to reduce BP. Alternative name is *arfonad*.

**Triple A**   *Quick Reference:* Refers to vascular surgical operation.
*Advanced Reference:* Term used to indicate an 'abdominal aortic aneurysm'.

**Trismus**   *Quick Reference:* Spasm of the jaw muscles.
*Advanced Reference:* May be due to inflammation from a tooth abscess, throat infection or irritation of the cells controlling the muscles of the jaw (lock jaw).

**Trocar**   *Quick Reference:* Sharp instrument used for piercing a body cavity.

*Advanced Reference:* Used in conjunction with a cannula which is a shorter hollow tube fitting over the trocar so that the sharp end protrudes. When the trocar and *cannula* have been introduced, the trocar is withdrawn and fluid, air, etc. allowed to escape through the cannula. Used for *hydrocele, pneumothorax, cystostomy,* etc.

**Trochanter**   *Quick Reference:* (troc-ant-er) Two large knobs at the upper end of the femur.

*Advanced Reference:* The lesser and greater trochanter, to which are attached various muscles acting on the hip.

**Trochlea(r)**   *Quick Reference:* (troc-lia) Pulley shaped.

*Advanced Reference:* The trochlea. Can refer to the trochlear nerve which is the fourth cranial nerve and supplies the superior oblique eye muscle or the area involving the frontal bone through which the tendon of the superior oblique eye muscle passes.

**Trouser graft**   *Quick Reference:* Synthetic vascular graft.

*Advanced Reference:* Y-shaped (inverted) synthetic vascular graft used to replace a portion of the aorta and femoral arteries.

**Trypsin**   *Quick Reference:* A digestive enzyme.

*Advanced Reference:* Trypsin converts protein into amino acids. Trypsinogen is secreted in the pancreas and is converted in the intestine into active trypsin.

**Tubal ligation**   *Quick Reference:* Surgical female sterilisation.

*Advanced Reference:* Involves interruption of fallopian tube continuity by excising a segment of each tube followed by ligation of each free end. May be done laparoscopically, open surgical method or involve clipping of the tubes so *patency* is lost.

**Tubercle**   *Quick Reference:* A small lump.

*Advanced Reference:* Usually refers to a prominence on a bone but also indicates the lesion produced by the *tuberculosis* (*TB*) micro-organism, *Mycobacterium tuberculosis.*

**Tuberculosis**   *Quick Reference:* Infectious disease caused by *Myobacterium tuberculosis.*

*Advanced Reference:* The disease process destroys the tissues involved, lungs being the most common but can manifest in numerous parts of the body. Acquired primarily via breathing. Treatment at one time was revolutionised by the discovery of streptomycin. Immunisation is with the Bacille Calmette Guerin (BCG) vaccine, made from an attenuated strain of *Myobacterium bovis.*

**Tuberosity**   *Quick Reference:* A protuberance on a bone.

*Advanced Reference:* The tibial tuberosity is a raised surface on the *tibia* and the radial tuberosity is a protuberance on the radial shaft into which the *tendon* of the *biceps* muscle inserts.

T

**Tube support** *Quick Reference:* Device for supporting anaesthetic tubing during surgery.

*Advanced Reference:* Designed to keep the tubing away from the patient's face, etc. and avoid kinking as well as facilitating necessary direction, tube supports either attach to the table end or slide under the table mattress.

**Tubigrip** *Quick Reference:* Type of cylindrical support bandage.

*Advanced Reference:* Supporting those type of bandage or dressing used as support following injury, post-operatively and intra-operatively for certain procedures.

**Tubocurarine** *Quick Reference:* Non-depolarising muscle relaxant.

*Advanced Reference:* Tubocurarine is the active principle of Curare, a South American arrow poison and original non-depolarising muscle relaxant used in anaesthesia. A pure alkaloid D-tubocurarine (DTC) was isolated in 1935. Also known as *tubarine*.

**Tubule** *Quick Reference:* Small tube.

*Advanced Reference:* The collecting and conveying tubules in the kidney medulla which convey urine to the kidney pelvis.

**Tulle gras** *Quick Reference:* (tul-grar) A net of pliant material impregnated with soft paraffin.

*Advanced Reference:* May also be mixed with ointment containing *anti-septic* or *antibiotic*. Used as a dressing for raw surfaces such as burns, scalds or ulcers.

**Tumour** *Quick Reference:* Any swelling.

*Advanced Reference:* Usually used to mean a *benign* or *malignant* growth. A new growth is called a *neoplasm*.

**Tunica** *Quick Reference:* A tunic or coat, covering.

*Advanced Reference:* The lining of a vessel, intima as with blood vessels.

**Tuohy** *Quick Reference:* (tu-e) Epidural needle.

*Advanced Reference:* Epidural needle with an oblique bevelled tip and 1-cm markings (Alfred Lee type) designed to indicate the depth of the *epidural* space.

**Turbinates** *Quick Reference:* Bones of the nasal cavity.

*Advanced Reference:* Three scroll-shaped bones, superior, middle and inferior, that help form the walls of the nasal cavity.

**Turgid** *Quick Reference:* Inflated, enlarged.

*Advanced Reference:* Indicates distention, congestion or being swollen.

**TUR hook** *Quick Reference:* Piece of equipment used in endoscopic genito-urinary (GU) procedures.

*Advanced Reference:* Intended to be a support for light cables, diathermy leads, irrigation tubing during TURP, etc. Commonly suspends from ceiling or operating light but designs are available that clamp to the table.

**TUR syndrome**   *Quick Reference:* Condition/syndrome sometimes found following TURP.

*Advanced Reference:* Due to absorption of irrigating fluid (glycine) via the open prostatic vessels. Causes IV overload and hyponatraemia due to the dilutional effect on the circulation. Signs and symptoms include bradycardia, hypotension, convulsions, confusion and dyspnoea.

**Tympanic membrane**   *Quick Reference:* (tim-pan-ic) The ear drum.

*Advanced Reference:* A greyish membrane which detects sound vibrations.

**Tympanoplasty**   *Quick Reference:* (tim-pan-o-plasty) Repair of the ear drum.

*Advanced Reference:* Generally any reconstructive operation on the middle ear with the intention of improving hearing.

**Typhus**   *Quick Reference:* An infection spread by lice.

*Advanced Reference:* Primarily a disease of dirt caused by *Rickettsiae.*

**Ulcer** *Quick Reference:* Chronic defect in the surface of skin or mucous membrane.

*Advanced Reference:* Can be due to many causes and occur in numerous sites, i.e. *gastric and duodenal ulcers* of the stomach, *leg ulcers* involved with varicose veins, *rodent ulcers* associated with tumour formation.

**Ulceration** *Quick Reference:* The formation of ulcer.

*Advanced Reference:* Ulceration defines the break in continuity with the tissue surface. This can occur due to pressure on the skin surface causing restricted blood flow and potential necrosis of the tissue. Ulceration can occur within the trachea due to direct and overpressure of the inflated endotracheal (ET) tube cuff.

**Ulcerative colitis** *Quick Reference:* Disease of the colon and rectum.

*Advanced Reference:* The condition involves inflammation of the large bowel and possible ulceration. Cause is unknown but theories range from infection, allergy and auto-immune reaction.

**Ulna** *Quick Reference:* The bone on the underside of the forearm connecting between the wrist and the humerus.

*Advanced Reference:* The ulna is one of the essential structures of the forearm along with the radius. Both bones give protection to the radial and ulnar artery that run parallel to the bone surface. The ulnar nerve is a branch of the brachial plexus which descends on the medial side of the upper arm to the elbow. It is one of the most prominent nerves in terms of injury and damage in relation to patient positioning on the operating table.

**Ultrasonic** *Quick Reference:* Sound waves which are beyond the upper range audible to humans.

*Advanced Reference:* Utilised in various forms with medical and diagnostic equipment, i.e. Electrical shock wave *electrical shock wave lithotripsy* (ESWL), ultrasound, etc.

**Ultrasonic washer** *Quick Reference:* A device used to clean debris from the surface of surgical instruments.

*Advanced Reference:* The device emits ultrasonic waves which create high ripples that strike the object at a fast-rate shaking off the debris.

**Ultrasound**   *Quick Reference:* The utilisation of ultrasonic waves to examine the interior of the body.

*Advanced Reference:* Also used therapeutically in the treatment of soft tissue pain and lithotripsy shock wave therapy to break up renal stones.

**Umbilical cord**   *Quick Reference:* (um-bill-i-cal) Cord which connects an unborn infant to its *placenta*.

*Advanced Reference:* The cord which supplies nourishment to the *foetus* and is composed mainly of two arteries and a vein plus vestigal structures surrounded by a membrane.

**Umbilicus**   *Quick Reference:* The navel.

*Advanced Reference:* Depression in the middle of the abdomen where the umbilical cord enters.

**Underwater seal drainage**   *Quick Reference:* Type of chest drain.

*Advanced Reference:* Used after chest surgery, the drain is inserted into the pleura as a way of equalising pressure with the atmosphere. Allowing air into the pleura would cause collapse of the lung. The tubing from the pleura connects to a further tubing whose end is placed under the surface of sterile water in a jar and so allows air, etc. to exit the pleura but no air to enter and cause lung collapse.

**Unit**   *Quick Reference:* Single item.

*Advanced Reference:* Quantity. Designates as a standard of measurement.

**Universal precautions**   *Quick Reference:* Infection control guidelines designed to protect workers from exposure to diseases spread by blood and certain body fluids.

*Advanced Reference:* Universal precautions apply to tissue, blood and other body fluids, e.g. semen and vaginal secretions. Formulated in America in 1987 by the Centre for Disease Control and Prevention and basically indicates that all patients should be treated as positive until proved negative.

**Uraemia**   *Quick Reference:* (you-rem-e-a) Excess of urea in the blood.

*Advanced Reference:* Results from defective function of the kidneys.

**Urea**   *Quick Reference:* End product of protein breakdown.

*Advanced Reference:* Urea is excreted in the urine. An excess in the blood is termed *uraemia*.

**Ureter**   *Quick Reference:* (your-eat-tor) Tube leading from the kidney to the bladder.

*Advanced Reference:* There are two ureters which are muscular tubes and convey urine from the kidney to the bladder. The term ureteric is used when making reference to the ureters, e.g. ureteric *catheter*.

**Ureterolithotomy**   *Quick Reference:* (your-eat-row) Surgical removal of a ureteric calculus.

*Advanced Reference:* Carried out if the stone is causing recurrent pain, causing complete blockage or infection. Involves exposure and excision of the ureter for direct removal of the stone.

**Urethra** *Quick Reference:* Tube carrying urine away from the bladder.

*Advanced Reference:* The urethra is longer in the male than female. One consequence being that males have better protection against cystitis than the female. *Urethritis* is inflammation of the urethra.

**Uric acid** *Quick Reference:* A normal constituent of urine.

*Advanced Reference:* Lithic acid. *Uricaemia* is the accumulation of uric acid in the blood. A build-up can lead to renal *calculi* formation.

**Urinary diversions** *Quick Reference:* Operation carried out to divert the ureters, usually due to complete bladder removal, contracted bladder or irreparable vesico-vaginal fistula.

*Advanced Reference:* Two of the most common procedures are *ureterosigmoidostomy* and *uretero-ileostomy*. In the former the ureters are transplanted into the sigmoid colon but this procedure has the disadvantage of ascending infection. The latter operation involves isolating a section of ileum and bringing it to the abdominal wall then implanting the ureters into this conduit and so creating an ileostomy for urine collection.

**Urine** *Quick Reference:* Fluid secreted by the kidneys.

*Advanced Reference:* Urine is stored in the bladder after production in the kidneys. It is 96% water and 4% solids, the most important being *urea* and *uric acid*. Urinalysis involves the bacteriological and chemical examination of urine.

**Urography** *Quick Reference:* X-ray examination of the urinary tract.

*Advanced Reference:* The examination is carried out with the use of contrast media (urograffin). Urogram involves a radiograph of the urinary tract. Other related procedures are cystography (bladder) and pyelography (kidney).

**Urology** *Quick Reference:* Branch of medicine dealing with the urinary tract and related structures.

*Advanced Reference:* Involves disease of the urinary tract in both sexes and especially those of the genital organs in males.

**Urticaria** *Quick Reference:* (hurt-te-care-ear) *Allergy* reaction signified by redness of the skin. Also referred to as nettle rash.

*Advanced Reference:* Redness is due mainly to *histamine*, which is released when tissue is injured etc causes capillaries to leak fluid. Signs and symptoms generally include redness, itching and burning sensation sometimes combined with blistering.

**Uterus** *Quick Reference:* Refers to the female womb.

*Advanced Reference:* Triangular shaped, hollow, muscular organ sited in the pelvis between the rectum and bladder.

**Uvula**   *Quick Reference:* Fleshy prolongation at the back of the mouth.

*Advanced Reference:* The uvula hangs down in the middle of the throat over the base of the tongue.

**U-wave**   *Quick Reference:* Positive deflection seen on an Electrocardiographical (ECG) recording.

*Advanced Reference:* A positive deflection but of low amplitude. Not always present and thought to represent slow repolarisation of minor muscle.

# V

**Vaccine** *Quick Reference:* (vax-seen) Vaccination. To introduce a substance usually by injection in order to confer *immunity*.

*Advanced Reference:* A modified *virus* or *bacterium* which provokes immunity but does not produce the disease itself. Vaccination is now used synonymously with **immunisation** and **inoculation**.

**Vagal-tone** *Quick Reference:* Indicates a level of activity in the parasympathetic nervous system.

*Advanced Reference:* Inhibitory control of the vagus nerve over heart rate and atrioventricular (AV) conduction.

**Vagina** *Quick Reference:* Lower part of the female reproductive tract.

*Advanced Reference:* A muscular passage lined with mucous membrane extending from the uterus to the exterior.

**Vaginal hysterectomy** *Quick Reference:* Surgical removal of the uterus via the vaginal route.

*Advanced Reference:* Classified as a subtotal procedure; involves removal of the body of the uterus leaving the cervix in place.

**Vagotomy** *Quick Reference:* Surgical division (or partial) of the vagus nerve.

*Advanced Reference:* The object of removing vagal nerve influence from the stomach is to reduce the secretion of acid. Selective (highly) vagotomy diminishes the gastric secretions but leaves the emptying mechanism of the stomach intact, whereas complete (truncal) vagotomy may be accompanied by a pyloroplasty or gastro-enterostomy to ensure emptying of the stomach.

**Vagus nerve** *Quick Reference:* Component of the *parasympathetic* nervous system.

*Advanced Reference:* Tenth cranial nerve is also called vagus. It carries autonomic fibres to the organs of the abdomen and thorax, supplies motor fibres to the oesophagus, larynx and *pharynx*, sensory fibres to the larynx, pharynx, tongue and ear.

**Valgus** *Quick Reference:* Bent, twisted outwards.

*Advanced Reference:* Abnormal position of a limb. Indicating away from the midline.

**Valium**   *Quick Reference:* A mild tranquilliser with mild muscle-relaxant properties.

*Advanced Reference:* A proprietary preparation of *benzodiazepine* which may be used as a skeletal-muscle relaxant.

**Vallecula**   *Quick Reference:* (val-ek-you-la) Any crevice or depression on the surface of an organ or structure.

*Advanced Reference:* A groove between the base of the tongue and the *epiglottis.*

**Valsalva's manoeuvre**   *Quick Reference:* A test of the baroreceptor reflex.

*Advanced Reference:* Involves the patient exhaling forcefully against a closed larynx resulting in an increased intrathoracic pressure. This leads to decreased venous return and in turn a reduction in cardiac output coupled with a fall in blood pressure (BP). The reduced baroreceptor discharge to the vasomotor centre then causes vasoconstriction and an increase in heart rate.

**Valve**   *Quick Reference:* A fold of membrane, e.g. heart valve.

*Advanced Reference:* A valve may consist of two or three flaps or folds attached to the vessel wall like pockets.

**Valvotomy**   *Quick Reference:* A surgical procedure involving incision into a valve.

*Advanced Reference:* Usually performed to correct a defect and allow effective opening. Removes fibrosed tissue which can affect the function of the valve, e.g. mitral valvotomy for mitral stenosis.

**Vancomycin**   *Quick Reference:* An antibacterial antibiotic.

*Advanced Reference:* Can be taken orally in the treatment of colitis or via intravenous (IV) infusion for endocarditis and other serious infections.

**Vaporiser**   *Quick Reference:* A piece of anaesthetic equipment which converts a fluid to a vapour.

*Advanced Reference:* A device that allows controlled vaporisation of liquid anaesthetic agents.

**Varices**   *Quick Reference:* (var-is-seas) Dilated friable veins, e.g. around the gastro-oesophageal junction.

*Advanced Reference:* Normally associated with life-threatening bleeding in patients with oesophageal varices.

**Varicocoele**   *Quick Reference:* (varic-o seal) Varicose swelling of the testicular veins.

*Advanced Reference:* If symptomatic, treated by surgery which involves excision of the effected veins.

**Varicose veins**   *Quick Reference:* Swollen or dilated veins especially in the legs.

*Advanced Reference:* Abnormal swelling of veins in the legs due to a weakness in the valves in the walls of the veins.

**Vascular** *Quick Reference:* Relating to blood vessels. Also a surgical speciality.
*Advanced Reference:* May also relate to blocked, injured or diseased arteries and veins.

**Vas deferens** *Quick Reference:* The duct of the testis.
*Advanced Reference:* It carries spermatozoa via the prostate to the urethra.

**Vasectomy** *Quick Reference:* Male sterilisation.
*Advanced Reference:* Division and tying off of the *vas deferens* usually carried out via an incision in the *scrotum*.

**Vasoconstriction** *Quick Reference:* Reflex widening or narrowing of blood vessels.
*Advanced Reference:* Selective constriction or dilatation of vessels that can change or compensate blood pressure.

**Vasomotor** *Quick Reference:* Indicates the vasomotor centre in the medulla oblongata.
*Advanced Reference:* Responsible for the regulation of BP and cardiac function via the *autonomic nervous system*.

**Vasopressin** *Quick Reference:* A natural body hormone secreted by the posterior lobe of the pituitary gland.
*Advanced Reference:* Also known as antidiuretic hormone or ADH.

**Vasopressor drugs** *Quick Reference:* Drugs that cause vasoconstriction.
*Advanced Reference:* These drugs are used to bring about vasoconstriction and/or increase the BP. One example would be adrenaline during resuscitation. Also, *adrenaline* in combination with lignocaine causes local vasoconstriction and so extends absorption time of the local anaesthetic (LA).

**Vasovagal attack** *Quick Reference:* Fainting. Also referred to as vagovagal, a reflex response.
*Advanced Reference:* Stimulation of the vagus nerve. A reflex action in which irritation of the larynx or trachea results in bradycardia. Vasovagal response generally causes a drop in BP, *bradycardia,* fainting, etc.

**Vasoxine** *Quick Reference:* A vasoconstrictor drug.
*Advanced Reference:* Used to raise BP. It is a preparation of methoxamine hydrochloride.

**Vector** *Quick Reference:* An animal carrying infective organism, e.g the mosquito in malaria.
*Advanced Reference:* An animal that carries organisms or parasites from one host to another. To the same species or cross species.

V

**Vecuronium**   *Quick Reference:* (vec-you-roam-eum) A skeletal-muscle relaxant. Norcuron.

*Advanced Reference:* A non-depolarising muscle relaxant administered by injection under general anaesthesia (GA) during surgery. Has a duration of action of 20–30 minutes and little effect on the cardiovascular system. Does not produce *histamine*. Secreted in the bile but only to a minor degree through the kidneys so is suitable in cases of renal failure.

**Veins**   *Quick Reference:* Blood vessels carrying deoxygenated blood. Many of which contain one-way valves.

*Advanced Reference:* A thin-walled vessel which carries blood from the capillaries back to the heart.

**Velosef**   *Quick Reference:* Proprietary antibiotic.

*Advanced Reference:* One of the cephalosporin group of antibiotics (cephradine) available as syrup, tablets or the more common in relation to theatres, powder for reconstitution.

**Vena cavae**   *Quick Reference:* The two largest veins in the body.

*Advanced Reference:* Comprises (i) the *superior vena cava* (SVC) into which blood drains from the head, neck, arms and chest and (ii) the *inferior vena cava* (IVC) which receives blood from the legs and abdomen. Both empty into the right atrium of the heart.

**Venepuncture**   *Quick Reference:* Transcutaneous puncture of a vein.

*Advanced Reference:* Correct term for cannulation, setting up an IV, etc.

**Venereal**   *Quick Reference:* Pertaining to a sexually transmitted disease (STD).

*Advanced Reference:* A disease transmitted by sexual activity.

**Venflon**   *Quick Reference:* Type of IV cannula.

*Advanced Reference:* A name that has almost become a term synonymous with cannula although actually a brand name. Available in a full range of sizes with an injection port.

**Ventilator**   *Quick Reference:* An artificial-breathing machine.

*Advanced Reference:* A piece of equipment used in hospitals to inflate the lungs by positive pressure.

**Ventolin**   *Quick Reference:* A bronchodilator to aid breathing.

*Advanced Reference:* Used in patients with asthma and other breathing problems and appears in many forms, the most popular being aerosol inhaler.

**Ventral**   *Quick Reference:* Refers to the lower surface of the body.

*Advanced Reference:* Relating to or situated at or close to the front of the body or anterior part of an organ.

**Ventricle**   *Quick Reference:* A small pouch or cavity.

*Advanced Reference:* A small cavity, e.g. the ventricles of the heart or in the brain.

**Ventro-**  *Quick Reference:* Prefix indicates, in front of.
*Advanced Reference:* A ventro-fixation involves stitching a retroverted uterus or other abdominal organ to the abdominal wall and a ventro-suspension is performed to correct displacement of the uterus.

**Venturi mask**  *Quick Reference:* Oxygen-delivery system.
*Advanced Reference:* Type of oxygen mask that utilises the Venturi principle. The concentration of oxygen can be varied from 24% to 50% utilising a selection of detachable injectors which along with set delivery rates provides a fixed percentage.

**Venturi (principle)**  *Quick Reference:* Physics of principle involving pressure and flow.
*Advanced Reference:* The Venturi principle relates to the Bernoulli effect involving the effect on pressure by flow through a constriction, in that the inclusion of a side-arm to a pipe or tubing, will involve the entrainment of fluid or gas causing a mixing of the two. This principle is utilised in the Venturi or Mix-O-Mask oxygen-delivery system which allows for precise percentage oxygen settings.

**Venule**  *Quick Reference:* A small venous branch.
*Advanced Reference:* Venuoles are very small vessels that collect blood from capillaries.

**Verapamil**  *Quick Reference:* A calcium-antagonist anti-arrhythmic drug.
*Advanced Reference:* Used to treat high BP, angina and arrhythmias. Available as Cordilox.

**Veriform**  *Quick Reference:* Worm-shaped structure.
*Advanced Reference:* Pertaining to the worm-shaped structure attached to the appendix.

**Vertebrae**  *Quick Reference:* Segment of the backbone.
*Advanced Reference:* There are 33 vertebrae of which the upper 24 are separate bones, the next 5 are fused to form the sacrum and the lowest 4 form the coccyx.

**Vertex**  *Quick Reference:* The crown of the head.
*Advanced Reference:* Position of the foetus when the crown of the head appears in the vagina first.

**Vesico-vaginal fistula**  *Quick Reference:* (ves-i-co) Pertaining to bladder and vagina.
*Advanced Reference:* An abnormal passage between the bladder and the vagina.

**Vestibule**  *Quick Reference:* An entrance, space. Going into.

*Advanced Reference:* The oral vestibule is the area of the mouth between the teeth and cheeks, i.e. entrance to the oral cavity.

**Viable**  *Quick Reference:* Capable of independent life.
*Advanced Reference:* The term applied to a foetus capable of living outside the womb after the 28th week of pregnancy.

**Villi**  *Quick Reference:* Small finger-like projections.
*Advanced Reference:* A small protrusion from the surface of a mucous membrane, e.g. the small intestine.

**Virulence**  *Quick Reference:* The power of a bacteria or virus to cause disease.
*Advanced Reference:* Can be measured by how many people the micro-organism infects and how quickly it spreads through the body.

**Virus**  *Quick Reference:* The smallest microbe that cannot be seen under a microscope.
*Advanced Reference:* A microbe that lives inside a host cell and uses the host to multiply. Viruses cause many diseases and are resistant to antibiotics.

**Viscera**  *Quick Reference:* (vis-sera) Organs within the body cavities.
*Advanced Reference:* Usually applies to the large internal organs, e.g. lungs, liver and intestines.

**Vitreous humour**  *Quick Reference:* Transparent fluid that fills the eye.
*Advanced Reference:* It is in fact jelly like and fills the posterior chamber of the eye between the *retina* and the lens.

**Vitro (in)**  *Quick Reference:* Means literally 'in glass'.
*Advanced Reference:* Term applied to artificial insemination, i.e. test-tube baby, fertilisation in the laboratory, etc., whereas *vivo (in)* indicates within the living animal.

**Vocal cords**  *Quick Reference:* Two folds of mucous membrane that lie in the *larynx*.
*Advanced Reference:* They can be relaxed or be made tense by the muscles of the larynx. When air is forced through, they vibrate and produce the voice.

**Volatile**  *Quick Reference:* Substance that has a tendency to evaporate easily.
*Advanced Reference:* Term applied to various anaesthetic-inhalation agents, such as *halothane, enflurane, isoflurane, sevoflurane, desflurane*, etc., all delivered to the patient via a *vaporiser*. To some extent all are modern-day ethers, although not in a chemistry sense, that have been improved in terms of hepatoxicity, cardiovascular effects, uptake and elimination from the body condition specific, etc.

**Voltarol**  *Quick Reference:* Non-steroidal anti-inflammatory drug (*NSAID*), e.g. diclofenac sodium.

*Advanced Reference:* A non-narcotic analgesic used to treat pain and inflammation. May be administered orally, by tablet or suppositories. Has a number of side effects including nausea, gastrointestinal disturbance and can produce rash and *asthma* symptoms.

**Volvulus**  *Quick Reference:* (vol-view-lus) Condition in which a loop of bowel twists around itself.

*Advanced Reference:* This twisting can lead to intestinal obstruction and cutting off of the blood supply.

**Vomiting**  *Quick Reference:* A reflex protective reaction of stomach contents.

*Advanced Reference:* The expulsion of stomach contents via the oesophagus and the mouth.

**Von Recklinghausen's**  *Quick Reference:* (disease) Hereditary disorder with fibrous swellings of nerves.

*Advanced Reference:* Referred to as neurofibromatosis. Patients with this condition may have these growths in their airway and can cause stridor or upper airway sounds.

**Von Willebrand's disease**  *Quick Reference:* Inherited coagulation disorder.

*Advanced Reference:* Involves the deficiency of a protein involved in platelet adhesion and carriage of factor VIII.

**Vulva**  *Quick Reference:* The external female genitalia.

*Advanced Reference:* Includes the mons pubis, the labia majora and minora, external urethral orifice and clitoris.

**Waldeyer's ring**  *Quick Reference:* (wall-ders) A circle of lymphoid tissue found at the entrance to the pharynx.

*Advanced Reference:* Specialised lymphoid tissue involving tonsils, adenoids and lingual tonsil and acts as the first line of defence against upper respiratory tract infections.

**Warfarin**  *Quick Reference:* (warf-a-rin)A compound that prevents the clotting of blood.

*Advanced Reference:* Works by counteracting vitamin K. Usually given orally in the treatment of deep vein thrombosis (DVT), pulmonary embolism, after vascular surgery and following the replacement of heart valves. Also used as a rat poison.

**Warming blanket**  *Quick Reference:* Broad term for equipment and various devices used to maintain patients temperature during surgery.

*Advanced Reference:* Various designs of under- and over-blankets are now used. The term warming blanket was used at one time to mainly indicate water blankets which were placed on the operating table under the patient with some designs having ripple facility. Most designs now utilise warm air flow as the heating method.

**Waterlow scale**  *Quick Reference:* Pressure sore prevention policy.

*Advanced Reference:* It is basically a risk assessment tool for pressure sore prevention based on risk factors which include build/weight, continence, skin type, mobility, sex/age, appetite and special risks, malnutrition, neurological deficit, surgery/trauma and medications. The patient is given a score for each and added together can provide a cumulative-risk status.

**Water manometer**  *Quick Reference:* Measuring scale used for central venous pressure (CVP).

*Advanced Reference:* Involves a drip set connected to a three-way tap at the junction of the patient line and the vertical manometer scale which reads in cmH$_2$O. When the tap is directed appropriately, backpressure causes a rise in fluid from the intravenous (IV) bag up the manometer limb and levels out at the pressure exerted by the patients CVP.

Importantly, the 0 (zero) on the manometer scale must be at a set level (right atrium) at all times for accurate readings. In between readings, the tap can be directed so that the apparatus functions as a standard IV line.

**Waters**   *Quick Reference:* Collection of various anaesthetic-related equipment named after or devised by the American anaesthetist R.M. Waters.

*Advanced Reference:* Known most significantly for the Waters circuit, known as the to-and-fro system which incorporated a soda-lime canister into the circuit for ***carbon dioxide*** ($CO_2$) absorption. Now widely used without the canister but still referred to as Waters. Also, the Waters oropharyngeal airway made of metal with a side-arm for attaching a gas supply.

**Water soluble**   *Quick Reference:* Indicates that a substance can be washed away with water or will dissolve into water.

*Advanced Reference:* There are a number of substances and medications which fall into this category, e.g. water-soluble lubricants, certain contrast mediums used during angiography, etc.

**Watt**   *Quick Reference:* SI unit of power.

*Advanced Reference:* Equal to 1 joule per second.

**Weal**   *Quick Reference:* Localised area of ***oedema***.

*Advanced Reference:* Commonly found on the skin and produces itching.

**Weaning**   *Quick Reference:* To wean. To reduce reliance upon.

*Advanced Reference:* Term used with regard to minimising the patient's reliance of artificial ventilation. Also referred to during the newborn's activity for breastfeeding and removal to normal feeding.

**Wedge pressure**   *Quick Reference:* Refers to pressure measured within the pulmonary arterial system.

*Advanced Reference:* Carried out with a CVP-type catheter (Swann–Ganz/flotation, etc.) inserted via a central vein and guided through the right atrium to the ventricle and to eventually wedge in a branch of the pulmonary artery. The pressure recorded represents left atrial filling pressure and so, left ventricular end-diastolic pressure.

**Wedge resection**   *Quick Reference:* Surgical excision of part of an organ.

*Advanced Reference:* Example would be resection of an ovary containing a cyst. Sometimes termed *wedge excision*.

**Welt**   *Quick Reference:* Raised ridge of skin.

*Advanced Reference:* Commonly caused by a blow or impact.

**Wenckebach phenomenon**   *Quick Reference:* Abnormal heart rhythm.

*Advanced Reference:* This involves the gradual increase in PR interval until a beat is missed.

**Wertheims procedure**   *Quick Reference:* (vert-himes) Type of hysterectomy.

*Advanced Reference:* Total hysterectomy, involving removal of uterus, fallopian tubes, ovaries, lymph glands, cervix and top portion of the vagina.

**Whiplash**  *Quick Reference:* Neck injury commonly associated with automobile accidents.

*Advanced Reference:* Happens during sudden acceleration or deceleration when the head may be jerked forwards or backwards flexing and extending the neck causing injury to the cervical spine and related muscles.

**Whipple's**  *Quick Reference:* Pancreatico-duodenectomy carried out due to *carcinoma* of the (head) of *pancreas*.

*Advanced Reference:* Removal of the carcinoma located at the head of the pancreas which also involves removal of the *duodenum*, part of the pyloric end of the stomach and part of the *common bile duct*. The free ends of these structures are then anastomosed separately to a loop of *jejunum*. If the tumour is inoperable and causing obstructive *jaundice*, this can be relieved by bypassing the site of obstruction, i.e. *anastomosis* between the gall bladder and jejunum or duodenum.

**White matter**  *Quick Reference:* Medullated and fibrous part of the brain and spinal column.

*Advanced Reference:* Parts of the brain and spinal cord composed mainly of nerve fibres.

**Whole blood**  *Quick Reference:* Term used to indicate a unit of blood that is complete in volume as when removed from the donor (plus anticlotting agents).

*Advanced Reference:* The term indicates the alternative to blood that has had volume (*plasma*) removed, i.e. 'packed-cells' or 'plasma-reduced blood' which is useful when volume replacement is not as critical or the entire objective.

**Willis (circle of)**  *Quick Reference:* Circular system of arteries at the base of the brain.

*Advanced Reference:* Blood is carried to the skull by the left and right carotid and basilar arteries. The communicating branches form a ring. This arrangement provides an alternative supply if one artery fails but the main function of the circle is to balance the pressure of blood delivered to the brain.

**Wilms' tumour**  *Quick Reference:* Malignant tumour of the kidney.

*Advanced Reference:* A nephroblastoma which occurs in children.

**Wiring**  *Quick Reference:* Term used in relation to orthopaedic surgery regarding bone fixation.

*Advanced Reference:* Usually made of stainless steel and used to fixate bone fragments. Also refers to wiring of jaw (mandible) fractures.

**Wolff–Parkinson–White syndrome**  *Quick Reference:* A cardiac conduction abnormality.

*Advanced Reference:* Involves impulses short-cutting to the ventricles and bypassing the atrioventricular (AV) node due to an abnormal conduction pathway between the atria and the ventricles. The electrocardiography (ECG) reveals a short PR-interval that is often incorporated within the QRS-complex. Sufferers can sometimes spontaneously go into supraventricular tachycardia or atrial fibrillation.

**Womb** *Quick Reference:* The uterus.

*Advanced Reference:* Lay term for the female uterus.

**Wound drain** *Quick Reference:* An item or piece of equipment used to drain fluids from a body cavity.

*Advanced Reference:* Utilised usually after surgery and can be passive or active. Examples are corrugated drain, sump drain, suction drain and underwater seal.

**Wright respirometer** *Quick Reference:* Device used to measure patients tidal and minute volumes.

*Advanced Reference:* Both electronic and mechanical versions are available and are usually sited within the expiratory side of the breathing system. For accuracy, the respirometer requires a minimum flow of usually 2 litres/min.

**Xenograft**   *Quick Reference:* (sen-o graft) A type of organ or tissue *graft*.
*Advanced Reference:* A graft carried out between different species.

**Xphoid**   *Quick Reference:* Sword shaped.
*Advanced Reference:* The xphoid process is the smallest of three parts of the sternum which articulates with the inferior end of the sternum and the seventh rib. Also referred to as the *xiphisternum*.

**X-rays**   *Quick Reference:* Also known as Roentgen rays.
*Advanced Reference:* Electromagnetic radiation of shorter wave length than ultraviolet rays and are capable of penetrating many substances as well as producing changes in living matter. Due to this ability to affect matter, protection from X-rays is a vital part of theatre safety during exposure and takes the form of *lead aprons*, thyroid protectors, screens and most valuable of all, distance, as there is a degree of scatter of the rays. Monitoring badges are worn by those in regular contact with X-rays and records exposure and absorption levels.

**Xylocaine**   *Quick Reference:* (sy-low-cane) *Local anaesthetic* (LA) agent.
*Advanced Reference:* Most commonly used LA agent also known as **lignocaine**. Can be used for **infiltration**, intravenous (*IV*), *topical* and in epidural/spinals. It has a rapid onset with an average duration of 1.5–2 hours and extended by the addition of **adrenaline**. Has toxic effects, if the maximum dose is exceeded. Also used as an **anti-arrythmic**.

**Xylocard**   *Quick Reference:* (sy-low card) Proprietary anti-arrhythmic drug.
*Advanced Reference:* Used to treat heartbeat irregularities, such as ventricular ectopics and after various forms of heart attack. Available in a pre-loaded syringe for infusion. It is a preparation of anhydrous lignocaine.

**Yankauer** *Quick Reference:* (yan-ker) Type of suction device.

*Advanced Reference:* A rigid plastic or metal suction device with fixed curved tip used in surgery (oral) and anaesthesia.

**Y-can** *Quick Reference:* Design of intravenous (IV) cannula.

*Advanced Reference:* Designed to have a main channel and side injection/infusion port. There are two versions: a one-way and two-way. The one-way has a main channel with all injections given via a remote flexible side arm. The two-way appears similar but allows for an IV via the main channel and the side arm to run an infusion simultaneously.

**Y-drip set** *Quick Reference: Bifurcated* drip set.

*Advanced Reference:* IV giving-set which allows for two fluids, e.g. blood and saline, to be infused simultaneously.

**Y-piece** *Quick Reference:* Bifurcated connection, etc.

*Advanced Reference:* Usually refers to Y-piece connections in *anaesthetic circuits* but can be a connection in suction tubing, etc.

**Y-plasty** *Quick Reference:* Surgical revision of a scar.

*Advanced Reference:* Utilises a Y-shaped incision to reduce scar contracture.

# Z

**Zadiks operation**   *Quick Reference:* (zad-icks) **Radical** excision of the nail bed.
*Advanced Reference*: Radical excision involves the permanent **ablation** of the nail and nail bed. Other procedures on the big toe include *wedge resection*.

**Zantac**   *Quick Reference: H₂ receptor-blocking agent.*
*Advanced Reference:* Alternative name is *ranitidine*. Inhibits gastric secretions. Used in premedication, given approximately 1 hour before induction of **anaesthesia**.

**Zinacef**   *Quick Reference:* (sin-a-sef) A proprietary broad-spectrum antibiotic.
*Advanced Reference:* A preparation of *cefuroxime* and produced in the form of a powder for reconstitution.

**Zinc oxide**   *Quick Reference:* Mild astringent used to treat skin rashes, etc.
*Advanced Reference:* Also used to impregnate bandages and sticking tape/plaster (zinc oxide tape).

**Zip**   *Quick Reference:* A surgical zip used to close the *abdominal cavity*.
*Advanced Reference:* During abdominal surgery where the two edges of the surgical incision cannot be approximated due to enlargement of abdominal contents a surgical zip can be used. The outer edges of the zip can be cut to the required shape, they are then stapled or sutured in place. A surgical zip is a temporary measure until abdominal swelling is reduced and the skin edges can be brought together.

**Zoster**   *Quick Reference:* Herpes zoster. Shingles.
*Advanced Reference:* Virus responsible for this disease, the same as that which causes chickenpox. After initial infection, lays dormant in the nerve cells and later in life can reappear and produces herpes zoster.

**Z-plasty**   *Quick Reference:* Term used to describe a type of incision.
*Advanced Reference:* It is in reality a procedure used for removing scar tissue or repairing deformity.

**Zygoma**  *Quick Reference:* (zi-goma) Or zygomatic bone, Facial bone which gives shape to the cheek.

*Advanced Reference:* The zygomatic arch is an extension of the skull that connects to the zygoma giving rise to the shape of the cheek. Often injured during trauma and requires surgical elevation.

**Zygote**  *Quick Reference:* (si-goat) A single fertilized cell.

*Advanced Reference:* The fertilized ovum. Formed from the fusion of male and female germ cells.

# Useful web sites

## Anaesthesia

www.aagbi.org
www.anaesthetist.com
www.aodp.org
www.nda.ox.ac.uk
www.oaa-anaes.ac.uk
www.virtual-anaesthesia-textbook.com

## Educational institutions

www.edgehill.ac.uk

## Government

www.chi.nhs.uk
www.doh.gov.uk
www.hsedirect.com
www.medical-devices.gov.uk
www.nelh.nhs.uk
www.skillsforhealth.org.uk

## Health matters

www.amershamhealth.com
www.cpsm.org.uk
www.health-secure.net
www.hpc-uk.org
www.hsj.co.uk
www.issm.org.uk
www.naasp.org.uk
www.natn.org.uk
www.news.bbc.co.uk/health
www.nice.org.uk
www.nmc-uk.org
www.nursingtimes.net
www.opps.co.uk

www.pain-talk.co.uk
www.patients.association.com
www.rcn.org.uk
www.resus.org.uk
www.skillstat.com
www.smtl.co.uk
www.specialistinfo.com
www.surgical-tutor.org.uk
www.yoursurgery.com

### Discussion groups

http://groups.yahoo.com/group/ORNursesDownUnder
http://groups.yahoo.com/group/sterile
http://groups.yahoo.com/group/theatrepractitioners
http://website.lineone.net/trainee.odp/

### Medical

www.americanheart.org
www.bma.org.uk
www.bnf.org
www.dental12.demon.co.uk
www.dentanet.org.uk
www.doctors.net.uk
www.gdc-uk.org
www.gpinfo.com
www.hcsa.com
www.merseydeanery.ac.uk
www.mps.org.uk
www.resus.org
www.roysocmed.ac.uk
www.the-mdu.uk

### Research

www.cochrane.dk
www.evidence.org

### Surgical items

www.bbraun.com
www.ethicon.com
www.jnj.com
www.mapronproducts.co.uk
www.medgate.co.uk
www.swann-morton.com
www.timesco.com

# Table of normal values

## Conversion factors

### Solutions
1% solution = 1g in 100ml

### Temperature
Centigrade to Fahrenheit    $F = C \times 9/5 + 32$
Fahrenheit to Centigrade    $C = F - 32 \times 5/9$

### Volumes
Pints to litres = multiply by 0.568
Litres to pints = multiply by 1.760

### Weight
Pounds to kilograms = multiply by 0.454
Kilograms to pounds = multiply by 2.205
(approximately 1 stone = 6 kg)

### Pressure
$100\,kPa = 1\,bar = 1\,atm = 15\,lb/in^2 = 760\,mmHg$

## Composition of air

Nitrogen = 78%
Oxygen = 21%
Carbon dioxide = 0.03%

## Respiratory values

Tidal volume (TV) = 600 ml
Respiratory rate (RR) = 12–15
Minute volume (MV) = TV × RR
Anatomical dead space = 2 ml/kg
Vital capacity = 5000 ml

Total lung capacity = 6000–7000 ml
Oxygen consumption at rest = 200–250 ml/min
Carbon dioxide production at rest = 200 ml/min
(based approximately on 70 kg weight)

## Blood gas/acid–base values

pH = 7.36–7.42
$PCO_2$ = 35–45 mmHg
$PO_2$ = 80–100 mmHg
$O_2$ saturation = 85–100%
Standard bicarbonate = 22–26 mmol/l
Base excess = ±3 mmol/l

## Body water

|  | Male | Female |
|---|---|---|
| Fluid intake (24 h) | 3000 ml | 2500 ml |
| Fluid output (24 h) | 3000 ml | 2500 ml |
| Total body water | 45 l | 30 l |
| Intracellular | 30 l | 18 l |
| Extracellular | 15 l | 12 l |
| (+intravascular and interstitial) | | |

## Haematological values

|  | Male | Female |
|---|---|---|
| Haemoglobin | 14–18 g/100 ml | 12–16 g/100 ml |
| Haematocrit | 42–52% | 37–47% |
| White cells | 4000–10,000 cells/mm$^3$ | |
| Platelets | 150,000–400,000 mm$^3$ | |

## Normal biochemical values

Sodium = 133–144 mmol/l
Potassium = 3.2–5.1 mmol/l
Chloride = 96–109 mmol/l
Bicarbonate = 18–29 mmol/l
Calcium = 2.1–2.65 mmol/l
Fasting sugar = 3.4–6.2 mmol/l

## Body temperature

(normal)    36.8 C
            98.4 F